D1192471

ANATOMY FOR

VINYASA FLOW
AND
STANDING POSES

RAY LONG, MD, FRCSC

bandha yoga publications

This book is intended as a reference volume only, not as a medical manual. It is not to be used in any manner for diagnosis or treatment of medical or surgical conditions. This book is also not intended to be a substitute for any treatment that may be or has been prescribed by your health care provider. If you suspect that you have a medical problem, consult your physician. Always, in your particular case, obtain medical clearance from your physician before beginning the practice of yoga or any other exercise program. Always practice yoga under the direct guidance and supervision of a qualified and experienced instructor. Working directly with a qualified yoga instructor can help to prevent injuries. The author, illustrators, editor, publisher and distributor specifically disclaim any responsibility or liability for injuries that may occur during the practice of yoga or any other exercise program.

Published by Bandha Yoga Publications
Plattsburgh, NY
www.bandhayoga.com

Copyright ©2010 Raymond A. Long, MD, FRCSC
All content, visual and textual, produced under the direction of Ray A. Long, MD, FRCSC

All rights reserved.

No part of this book may be reproduced, stored in a retrieval system, or transmitted by any means, electronic, mechanical, photocopying, recording, or otherwise, without written permission from the publisher.

Mat Companion® is a registered trademark.

Distributed by Greenleaf Book Group LLC

For ordering information or special discounts for bulk purchases, please contact
Bandha Yoga Publications at 8908 Center Pointe Drive, Baldwinsville, NY 13027, 518.578.3720

Design and composition by Greenleaf Book Group LLC
Cover design by Greenleaf Book Group LLC
Front and back cover illustrations by Kurt Long, BFA   www.kurtlong.net
Computer Graphics Technical Director: Chris Macivor
Sanskrit calligraphy and border painting: Stewart Thomas   www.palmstone.com
Editor: Eryn Kirkwood, MA, RYT   www.barrhavenyoga.com

ISBN 13: 978-1-60743-943-1

Part of the Tree Neutral™ program, which offsets the number of trees consumed in the production and printing of this book by taking proactive steps, such as planting trees in direct proportion to the number of trees used: www.treeneutral.com

Printed in Canada on acid-free paper

10 11 12 13 14 15   10 9 8 7 6 5 4 3 2 1
First Edition

CONTENTS

INTRODUCTION

THE MAT COMPANION SERIES IS DESIGNED TO ASSIST YOU IN UNDERSTANDING the functional anatomy of yoga. Although all yoga poses are interrelated, for learning purposes we have subdivided them into categories according to their general form. This first book of the series shows how to combine Western scientific knowedge with the practice of Vinyasa Flow and the standing poses. In Vinyasa we repeat a foundational series of postures that encircle individual asanas from the other pose categories. This vigorous and aerobic practice combines breathing and body movement to produce heat, warming up the muscles, tendons, and ligaments and generating a detoxifying sweat. Practicing Vinyasa in a heated room enhances these effects. In the first part of this book, we discuss the practical application of Western science to Vinyasa Flow.

Following the Vinyasa portion of the book are the standing poses. Learning Hatha Yoga begins with these fundamental postures, which stretch and strengthen the muscles of the lower extremities and open the hips and pelvis. As a result of this practice, activities of daily living, such as standing and walking, feel comfortable and easy. Working the muscles and joints of the lower extremities also stimulates the nerve centers that supply this region, increasing electrical activity in the lumbosacral plexus. This increased electrical activity in turn illuminates the first and second chakras of the subtle body, aiding to remove energetic blockages that develop throughout our lifetime. It is this combination of biomechanical, physiological, and energetic processes that differentiate yoga from other forms of physical activity.

HOW TO USE THIS BOOK

Practicing yoga is like passing through a series of doors, with each door revealing new possibilities in the poses. The key to unlocking the first door is understanding the joint positions. This understanding can be used to identify the muscles that create the form of the pose and those that stretch. The key to positioning the joints is engaging the correct muscles. This begins with the prime movers. Engage the prime movers and the bones will align. The key to deepening the asanas is using your understanding of physiology to lengthen the muscles that stretch in the pose. Focus on these keys and the postures will automatically fall into place and manifest the beneficial effects of yoga. These include improved flexibility, heightened awareness, a sense of well-being, and deep relaxation.

The Mat Companion series is a set of modular books. Each book focuses on a specific pose category and contains the following:

- **The Key Concepts:** a description of biomechanical and physiological principles with applications for specific poses.
- **The Bandha Yoga Codex:** a simple five-step process that can be used to improve your flexibility, strength, and precision in the asanas.
- **The Pose Section:** a detailed description of the individual postures.
- **Movement Index:** explanations of body movement and tables listing the muscles associated with each movement.
- **Anatomy Index:** a visual listing of bones, ligaments, and muscles (showing the origins, insertions, and actions of each).
- **Glossary of Terms**
- **Sanskrit Pronunciation and Pose Index**
- **English Pose Index**

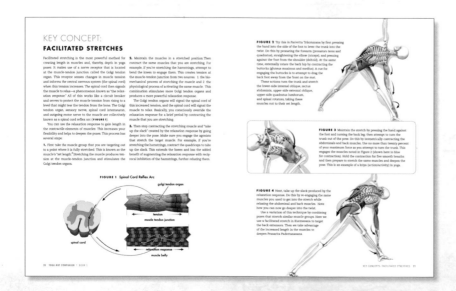

FIGURE 1 The Key Concepts show you how to apply biomechanics and physiology to your poses. Read this section first and return here often to refresh your knowledge.

FIGURE 2 The opening page for each pose illustrates the basic joint actions and positions of the body for that particular asana. Sanskrit and English names are provided for each posture. Use this page to assist you in learning the basic form of the pose and other concise details.

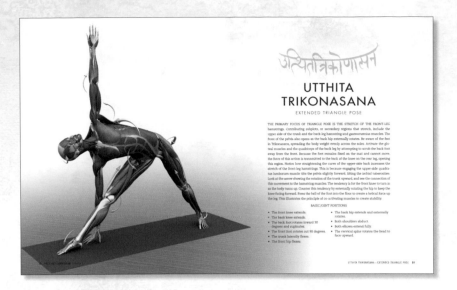

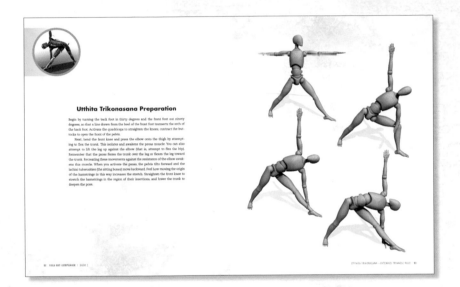

FIGURE 3 Use the preparatory section as a guide for how to enter the pose. If you are new to yoga or feel a bit stiff, use one of these modifications for your practice. In general the preparatory poses affect the same muscle groups as the final asana. You will benefit from the pose no matter which variation you practice.

FIGURE 4 Each pose comes with a series of steps for engaging the muscles that position the joints, concluding with a summary of the muscles that stretch. Muscles that contract are colored different shades of blue (with the prime movers deep blue), and those that stretch are red. Use the pose section to master the anatomy of any given asana.

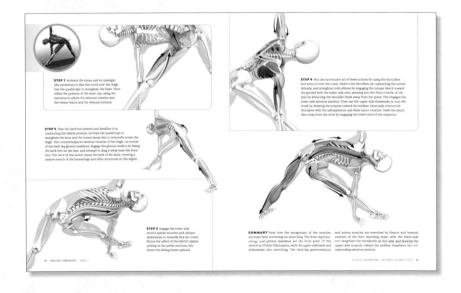

PRACTICE GUIDELINES

One of my favorite teachers, Professor Norm Fryman at Parson's School of Design, began his course by identifying three key attributes necessary for success in any endeavor. They are **common sense**, **discipline**, and **attention to detail**. Here are some suggestions on how to apply these attributes to your yoga practice:

1. Common Sense. Don't force yourself into a pose. In many yoga postures, joints can be taken to the extremes of their range of motion. Forcing the body into a position can injure the cartilage, ligaments, and muscles surrounding the joints. The Mat Companion series provides guidelines on how to use physiology to safely dissolve blockages and increase joint mobility. Use these guidelines to design your practice. Applying your knowledge of physiology rather than forcing yourself into the pose is akin to the ancient Chinese proverb, "If you have difficulty reaching your goal, keep the goal, but change your strategy."

2. Discipline. Yoga is about freedom—freedom of movement, thoughts, and energetic flow. Therefore, use discipline in moderation. Balance intensity with consistency. Regular practices of shorter duration are superior to high-intensity binges. Short and consistent practice integrates yoga into your life and produces long-lasting shifts and openings of energetic channels.

A practical way to combine modern technology and yoga is to use a timer. In fact, yoga master B.K.S. Iyengar often uses a stopwatch when practicing his poses. I have found this to be a particularly valuable tool, as it allows me to work each side of the body evenly. Using a timer also sets a limit on the asana (for example, 30 seconds). When the bell chimes, I'm finished with that pose and I don't think about it anymore. The timer is like a guru.

Another way to apply discipline to your practice is to take a moment to reflect on your session immediately after Savasana, or the final relaxation. Consider what went well and how you have improved; then leave it. Yoga instructors can use this same technique after teaching a class. This short reflection helps to consolidate the training session into your neural circuitry. Remember that the unconscious mind integrates your hard work into the body between sessions. Conscious reflection links your practice to the unconscious and multiplies this effect.

3. Attention to Detail. Art historian Aby Warburg once said, "God is in the details." When practicing Hatha Yoga with precise alignment, the body becomes the vehicle to union. As we breathe and move through the poses, chemical changes take place that produce a feeling of well-being and relaxation. Our drishti, or focus, combines with these chemical changes to quiet and calm the mind. The Mat Companion series provides a road map of muscles that activate and stretch and a step-by-step sequence of cues that you can apply in each asana. If you concentrate your drishti on the muscles that position the joints, your postures and alignment will improve and your state of mind will, too.

KEY
CONCEPTS

KEY CONCEPT
AGONIST/ANTAGONIST RELATIONSHIPS: RECIPROCAL INHIBITION

Typically, agonist/antagonist relationships involve muscles contracting and relaxing on opposite sides of a joint, creating a biomechanical Yin/Yang. One muscle contracts to move the joint in a certain direction while another opposes that movement and stretches during this action. For example, when the knee extends, the contracting quadriceps are the agonist muscles and the stretching hamstrings are the antagonists. Similarly, when the knee flexes, the hamstrings are the agonist muscles and the quadriceps are the antagonists. Joint movement in response to muscle contraction is a biomechanical event that is coupled with a physiological event—reciprocal inhibition. When the brain signals an agonist muscle to contract, it simultaneously signals the antagonist muscle to relax. This is a *physiological* Yin/Yang. Understanding the major agonist/antagonist relationships is one key to doing yoga poses well. Accordingly, it is important to learn the muscles and their actions. We illustrate these relationships for you throughout the Mat Companion series.

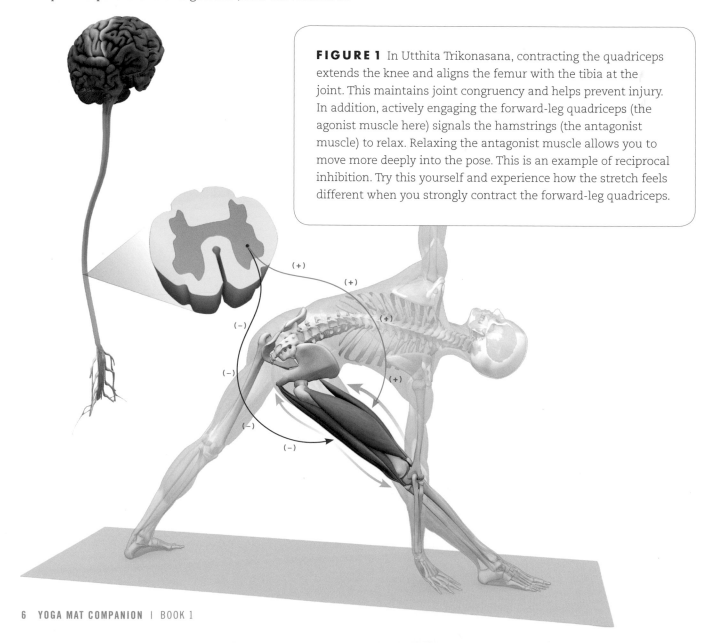

FIGURE 1 In Utthita Trikonasana, contracting the quadriceps extends the knee and aligns the femur with the tibia at the joint. This maintains joint congruency and helps prevent injury. In addition, actively engaging the forward-leg quadriceps (the agonist muscle here) signals the hamstrings (the antagonist muscle) to relax. Relaxing the antagonist muscle allows you to move more deeply into the pose. This is an example of reciprocal inhibition. Try this yourself and experience how the stretch feels different when you strongly contract the forward-leg quadriceps.

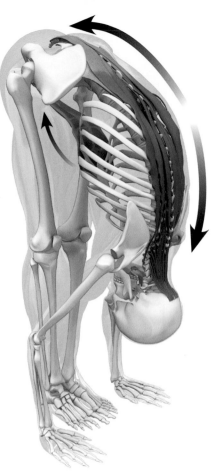

◀ FIGURE 2 In Uttanasana, the rectus abdominis flexes the trunk and signals its antagonist muscles, the erector spinae and quadratus lumborum, to relax. Engage this muscle in forward-bending poses to deepen the stretch of the antagonist back extensors.

▶ FIGURE 3 In Utthita Parsvakonasana, the psoas is the agonist muscle that flexes the hip and tilts the pelvis forward (anteversion). When the psoas contracts, the brain signals its antagonist muscle, the gluteus maximus (the main hip extensor), to relax into the stretch.

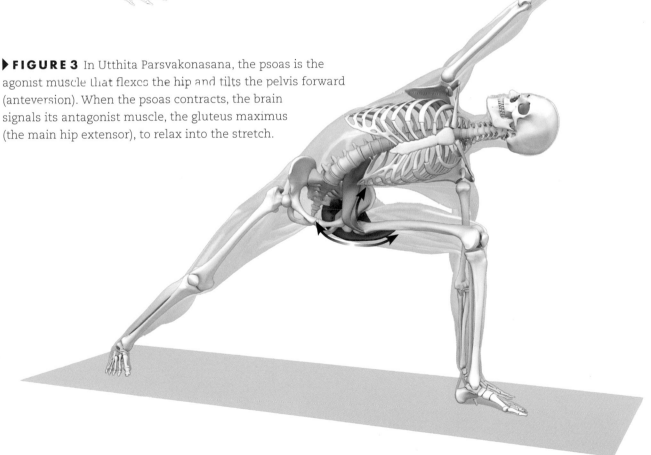

KEY CONCEPT
KEY MUSCLE ISOLATIONS

Muscles position the joints in the pose and align the bones. Although we can use gravity and other forces to attain the general shape of the asana, activating certain muscles provides precision. Use your muscles to sculpt the postures by isolating the "prime movers" of the joints—the muscles that produce the major joint actions. Here are some cues for engaging key muscles in the standing poses. You can also use visualization. Look at the images in this book and then visualize the individual muscles activating in the pose.

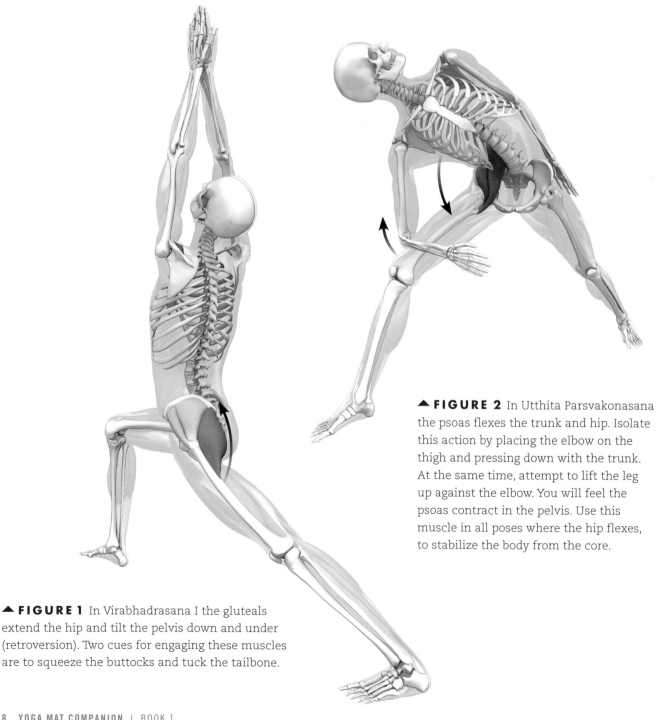

▲ **FIGURE 2** In Utthita Parsvakonasana the psoas flexes the trunk and hip. Isolate this action by placing the elbow on the thigh and pressing down with the trunk. At the same time, attempt to lift the leg up against the elbow. You will feel the psoas contract in the pelvis. Use this muscle in all poses where the hip flexes, to stabilize the body from the core.

▲ **FIGURE 1** In Virabhadrasana I the gluteals extend the hip and tilt the pelvis down and under (retroversion). Two cues for engaging these muscles are to squeeze the buttocks and tuck the tailbone.

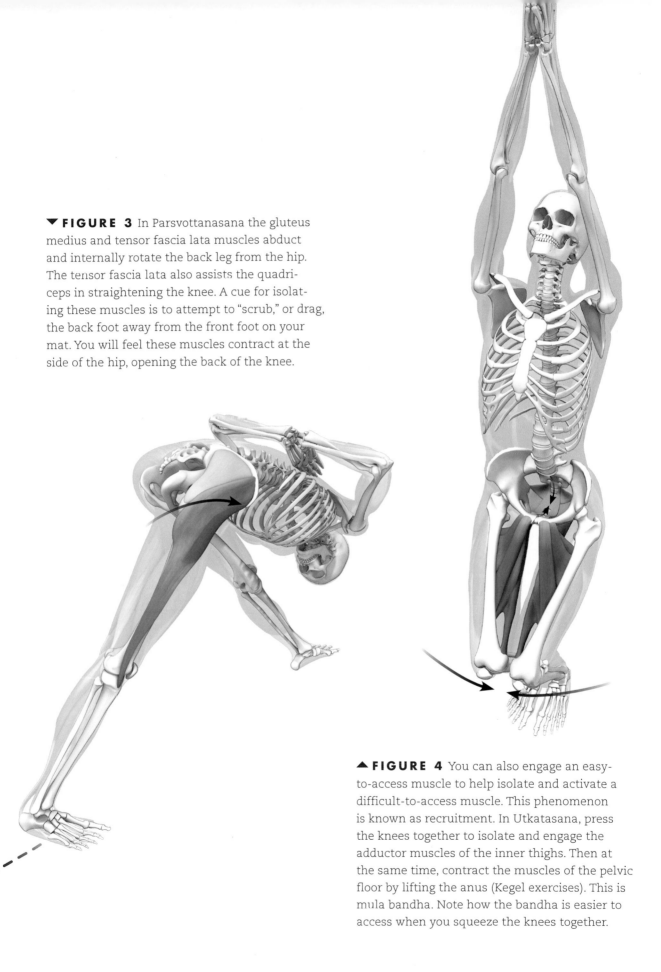

▼ **FIGURE 3** In Parsvottanasana the gluteus medius and tensor fascia lata muscles abduct and internally rotate the back leg from the hip. The tensor fascia lata also assists the quadriceps in straightening the knee. A cue for isolating these muscles is to attempt to "scrub," or drag, the back foot away from the front foot on your mat. You will feel these muscles contract at the side of the hip, opening the back of the knee.

▲ **FIGURE 4** You can also engage an easy-to-access muscle to help isolate and activate a difficult-to-access muscle. This phenomenon is known as recruitment. In Utkatasana, press the knees together to isolate and engage the adductor muscles of the inner thighs. Then at the same time, contract the muscles of the pelvic floor by lifting the anus (Kegel exercises). This is mula bandha. Note how the bandha is easier to access when you squeeze the knees together.

KEY CONCEPT
KEY CO-ACTIVATIONS

The ancient Chinese book of wisdom, the *I Ching*, has a hexagram devoted to the practice of yoga entitled "Keeping Still." To paraphrase the Wilhelm translation, "Movement posits stillness as an alternative." We move the body to position it in the postures, but ultimately we seek stillness and stability in our asanas. Co-activation of muscles is one way to achieve this quietude. There are many ways to perform co-activation, but all involve simultaneously contracting two or more muscles. For example, we can stabilize the pelvis by simultaneously contracting the psoas of the forward leg and the gluteus maximus of the rear leg in a standing pose. Stillness in the pelvis is then transmitted to the rest of the body (Fig. 1).

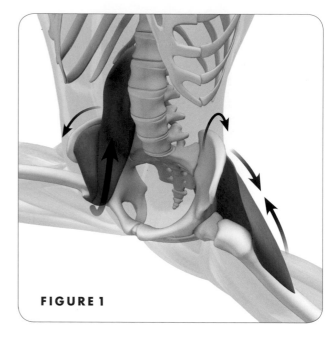

FIGURE 1

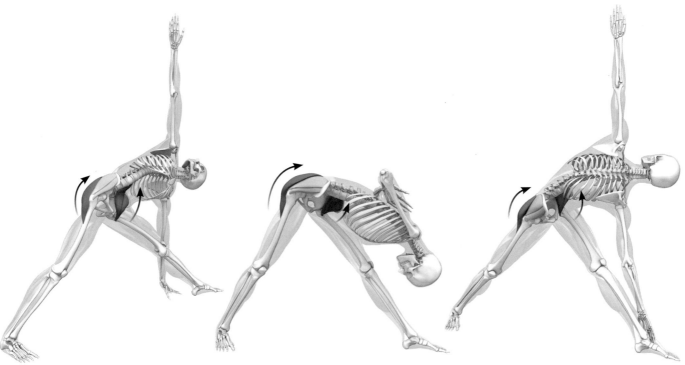

FIGURE 2 These images illustrate the dynamic process of co-activating the psoas and gluteus maximus using a series of standing poses that progressively turn the pelvis. You can sequence asanas in this way to awaken conscious control of these two core muscles—particularly the psoas. This newfound awareness allows you to directly contract these muscles in other pose categories, deepening trunk flexion and improving stability.

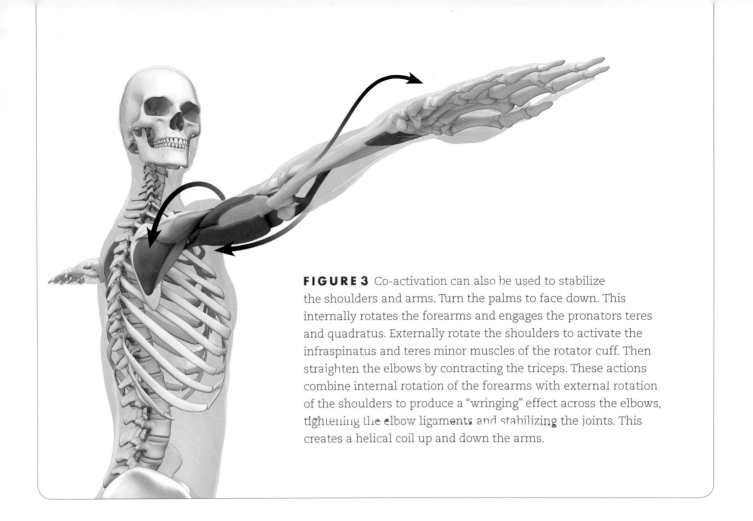

FIGURE 3 Co-activation can also be used to stabilize the shoulders and arms. Turn the palms to face down. This internally rotates the forearms and engages the pronators teres and quadratus. Externally rotate the shoulders to activate the infraspinatus and teres minor muscles of the rotator cuff. Then straighten the elbows by contracting the triceps. These actions combine internal rotation of the forearms with external rotation of the shoulders to produce a "wringing" effect across the elbows, tightening the elbow ligaments and stabilizing the joints. This creates a helical coil up and down the arms.

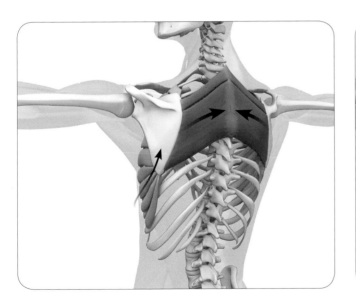

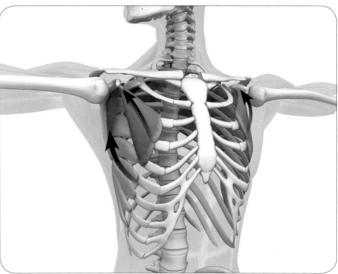

FIGURE 4 You can co-activate the accessory muscles of breathing to expand the ribcage, open the chest, and improve lung ventilation. Begin by contracting the rhomboids to draw the shoulder blades toward the spine. This stabilizes the scapulae and opens the chest. Maintain this position and then engage the pectoralis minor. You can isolate this muscle by attempting to roll the shoulders forward. The rhomboids will prevent the shoulders from moving, so the force of engaging the pectoralis minor is transmitted to its origin on the ribcage, lifting it. Activate the serratus anterior to expand the chest further. You will notice the breath deepening.

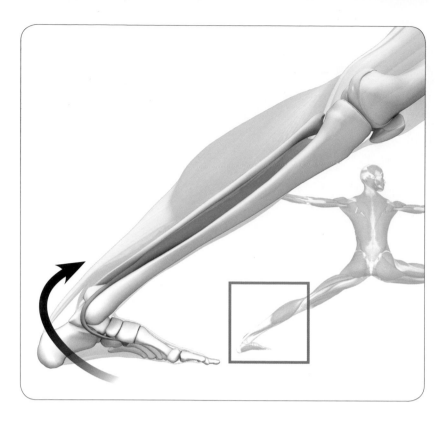

FIGURE 5 The foot and ankle are your connection to the earth in the standing poses. Use co-activation of muscles to stabilize this foundation. Turn the foot in and lift the arch by contracting the tibialis posterior. This muscle also bridges the two bones of the lower leg (the tibia and fibula), stabilizing the ankle joint. Begin by activating the tibialis posterior, and then engage its antagonist muscle group, the peroneus longus and brevis (located on the outside of the lower leg). To isolate the peronei, press the ball of the foot into the mat. Feel how co-contracting this agonist/antagonist group stabilizes the lower leg, ankle, and foot.

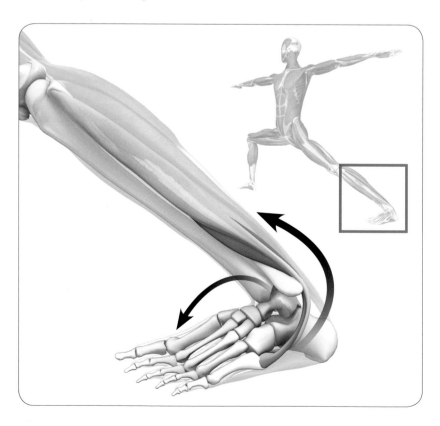

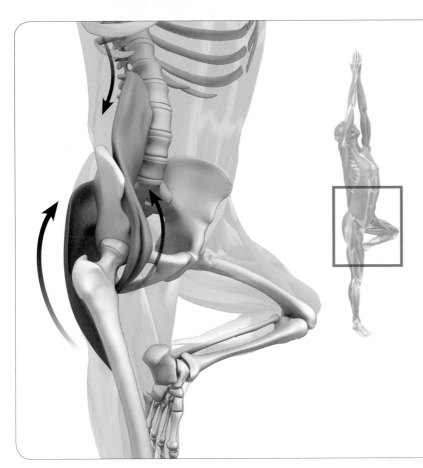

FIGURE 6 Co-contraction of the psoas and gluteus maximus stabilizes the pelvis from front to back in one-legged balancing poses. Visualize these muscles engaging during your practice.

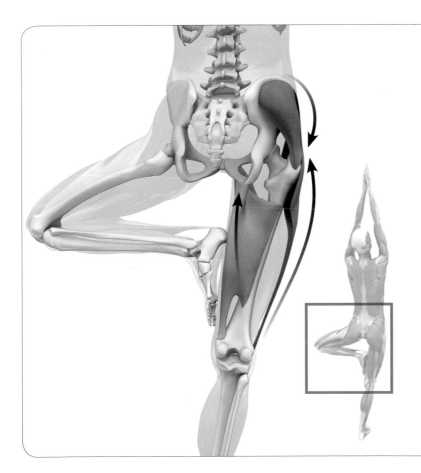

FIGURE 7 Co-contraction takes place automatically when we stand on one leg, as in Tree Pose. The gluteus medius and tensor fascia lata are abductor muscles typically used to draw the hip away from the midline. However, these muscles also pull downward on the ilium bone of the pelvis when we stand on one leg. If they didn't engage, the pelvis would shift over to the standing-leg side and we would lose balance. You can feel the tensor fascia lata and gluteus medius contracting by placing one hand on the outside of the hip in Vrksasana. In addition, the adductor muscles on the inner thighs co-contract to further stabilize the pelvis and hip. Visualize these muscles to gain awareness of this action.

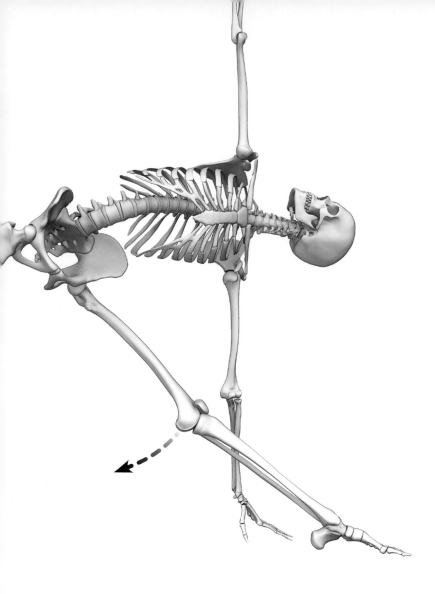

FIGURE 8 We are sometimes instructed to "hug the thigh bone" in a yoga class. This is an example of co-contraction. You can use a series of cues that isolate the different muscles surrounding a bone in order to achieve this effect. Apply this technique to correct hyperextension of the knee. Begin by isolating the hamstrings. The cue for this is to slightly bend the knee and attempt to "scrub," or drag, the front foot toward the back, as shown. The mat will prevent the foot from moving, but the hamstrings will engage. The hamstrings are knee flexors and contracting them prevents hyperextension. Then, maintaining tension in these muscles, engage the quadriceps to straighten the knee. From this image you can see that this agonist/antagonist muscle group, the hamstrings and quadriceps, surrounds the femur and crosses the knee joint. Co-contracting these muscles creates the "hug" that we sometimes hear about and prevents hyperextension of the knee in the pose.

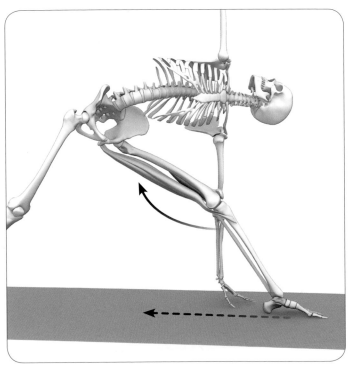

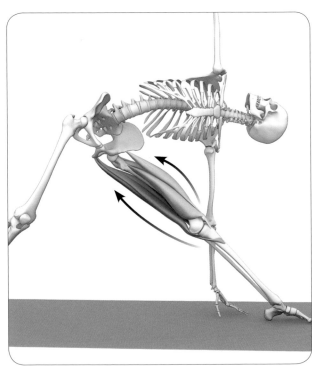

Bandha is a Sanskrit word that refers to a "lock" or "stabilizer." You can co-contract muscles to create locks or bandhas throughout the body in yoga poses. For example, in Parivrtta Parsvakonasana we turn the upper body in one direction and the lower body in the other.

Consciously engage the muscles that turn the trunk, such as the latissimus dorsi, posterior deltoid, and supraspinatus and infraspinatus muscles of the shoulder. Do this by pressing the elbow onto the knee to rotate the chest. Then at the same time, contract the gluteus maximus of the back leg to externally rotate the hip. Feel how these two actions combine to form a wringing effect across the torso, deepening and stabilizing the pose. This is an example of a bandha.

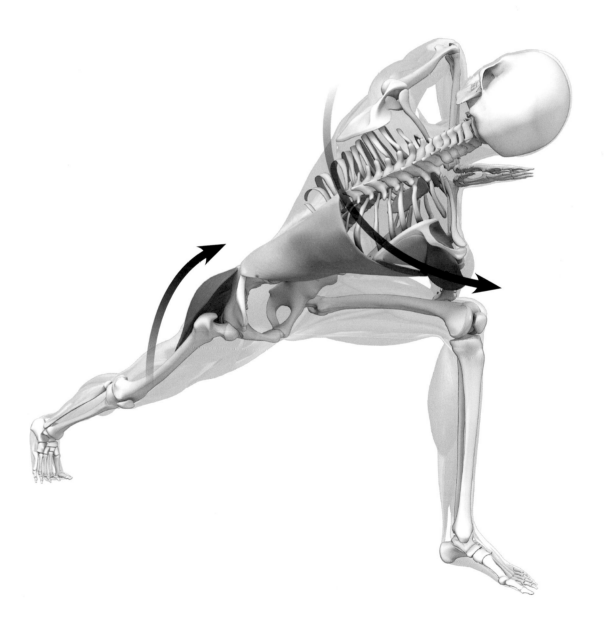

KEY CONCEPT
FACILITATED STRETCHES

Facilitated stretching is the most powerful method for creating length in muscles and, thereby, depth in yoga poses. It makes use of a nerve receptor that is located at the muscle-tendon junction called the Golgi tendon organ. This receptor senses changes in muscle tension and informs the central nervous system (the spinal cord) when this tension increases. The spinal cord then signals the muscle to relax—a phenomenon known as "the relaxation response." All of this works like a circuit breaker and serves to protect the muscle tension from rising to a level that might tear the tendon from the bone. The Golgi tendon organ, sensory nerve, spinal cord interneuron, and outgoing motor nerve to the muscle are collectively known as a spinal cord reflex arc (**FIGURE 1**).

You can use the relaxation response to gain length in the contractile elements of muscles. This increases your flexibility and helps to deepen the poses. This process has several steps:

1. First take the muscle group that you are targeting out to a point where it is fully stretched. This is known as the muscle's "set length." Stretching the muscle produces tension at the muscle-tendon junction and stimulates the Golgi tendon organs.

2. Maintain the muscles in a stretched position. Then contract the same muscles that you are stretching. For example, if you're stretching the hamstrings, attempt to bend the knees to engage them. This creates tension at the muscle-tendon junction from two sources: 1. the biomechanical process of stretching the muscle and 2. the physiological process of contracting the same muscle. This combination stimulates more Golgi tendon organs and produces a powerful relaxation response.

The Golgi tendon organs will signal the spinal cord of this increased tension, and the spinal cord will signal the muscle to relax. Basically, you consciously override the relaxation response for a brief period by contracting the muscle that you are stretching.

3. Then stop contracting the stretching muscle and "take up the slack" created by the relaxation response by going deeper into the pose. Make sure you engage the agonists that stretch the target muscle. For example, if you're stretching the hamstrings, contract the quadriceps to take up the slack. This extends the knees and has the added benefit of augmenting the relaxation response with reciprocal inhibition of the hamstrings, further relaxing them.

FIGURE 1 Spinal Cord Reflex Arc

Golgi tendon organ

tension

muscle-tendon junction

spinal cord

relaxation response

muscle belly

FIGURE 2 Try this in Parivrtta Trikonasana by first pressing the hand into the side of the foot to lever the trunk into the twist. Do this by pronating the forearm (pronators teres and quadratus), straightening the elbow (triceps), and pressing against the foot from the shoulder (deltoid). At the same time, externally rotate the back hip by contracting the buttocks (gluteus maximus and medius). A cue for engaging the buttocks is to attempt to drag the back foot away from the front on the mat.

These actions turn the trunk and stretch the lower-side internal oblique, rectus abdominis, upper-side external oblique, upper-side quadratus lumborum, and spinal rotators, taking these muscles out to their set length.

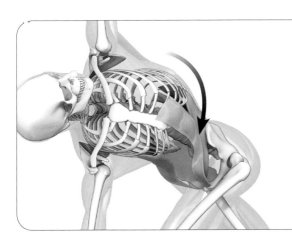

FIGURE 3 Maintain the stretch by pressing the hand against the foot and turning the back leg; then attempt to turn the trunk out of the pose. Do this by isometrically contracting the abdominals and back muscles. Use no more than twenty percent of your maximum force as you attempt to turn the trunk. This engages the muscles that were illustrated as stretching in Figure 2 (shown here in blue for contraction). Hold the contraction for five smooth breaths and then prepare to stretch the same muscles and deepen the pose. This is an example of a kriya (action/activity) in yoga.

FIGURE 4 Next, take up the slack produced by the relaxation response. Do this by re-engaging the same muscles you used to get into the stretch while relaxing the abdominal and back muscles. Note how you can now go deeper into the twist.

Use a variation of this technique by combining poses that stretch similar muscle groups. For example, on the next page, we illustrate using a facilitated stretch in Kurmasana to target the back extensors. Then we take advantage of the increased length in the muscles to deepen Prasarita Padottanasana.

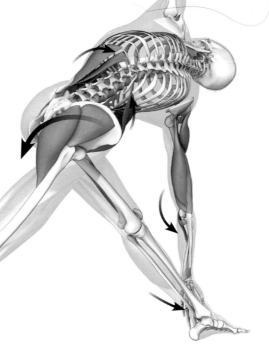

FIGURE 5 Place the arms under the legs in Kurmasana (Tortoise Pose). Engage the quadriceps to straighten the knees. This will hold the arms and trunk in flexion and is an example of connecting the upper and lower extremities. Contract the biceps to maintain a slight bend in the elbows to protect them against hyperextension.

Flexing the trunk takes the erector spinae and quadratus lumborum out to their set length, stretching these muscles and creating tension at the muscle-tendon junction. This is the first part of the facilitated stretch.

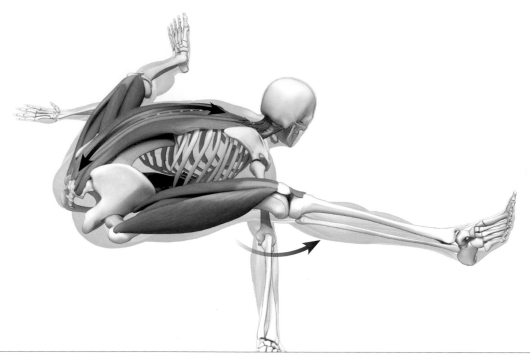

FIGURE 6 Now, attempt to arch the back and sit up (while holding your trunk in flexion with the quadriceps). This eccentrically contracts the spine extensors and recruits more Golgi tendon organs to fire. Maintain your attempt to arch the back for five to eight breaths, and then activate the rectus abdominis to flex the trunk (this produces reciprocal inhibition of the back extensors, relaxing them). Contract the quadriceps to straighten the knees and press down on the arms, deepening the pose. Come out and take Dandasana for a few moments to balance this intense stretch with a gentle contraction of the back extensors.

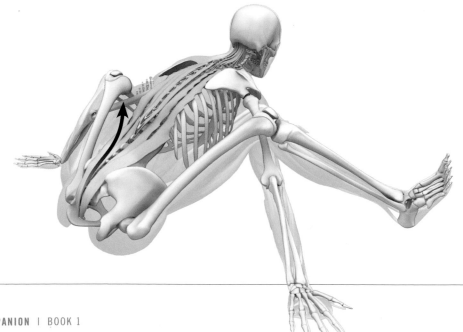

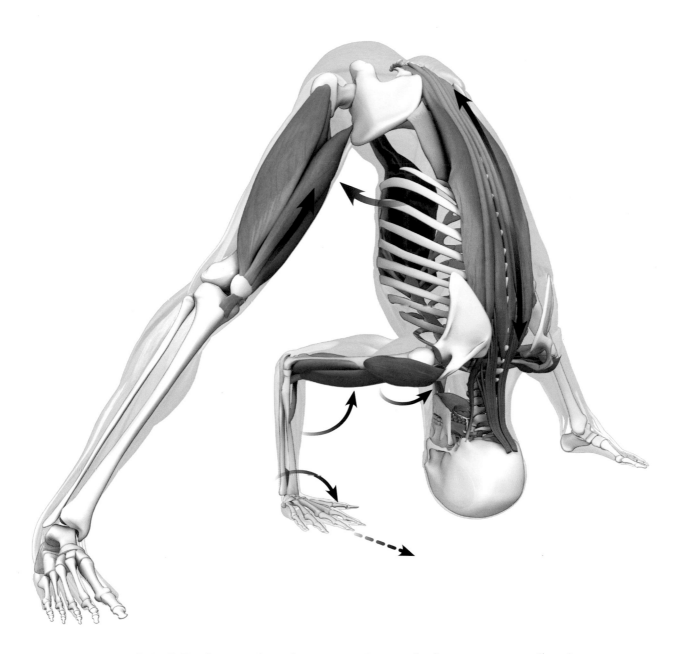

FIGURE 7 Take Prasarita Padottanasana. Pronate the forearms to press the palms into the mat, fixing them there. Then bend the elbows by engaging the biceps. At the same time, attempt to "scrub" the hands forward, as if you were going to raise the arms overhead. This activates the anterior deltoids. Squeeze the abdomen and straighten the knees by contracting the quadriceps. Note how preparing the back extensors with a facilitated stretch in Kurmasana allows you to go deeper into Prasarita Padottanasana.

THE BANDHA YOGA CODEX

EACH YOGA POSTURE HAS ITS OWN UNIQUE FORM AND FUNCTION. MUSCLES THAT engage in one posture may be stretching in another. For this reason it helps to have a road map for navigating your way to the optimal pose. Better still is the ability to create your own road map. The Bandha Yoga Codex shows you how to do this.

There are five elements to every asana. These are the joint positions, the muscles that engage to produce these positions, the muscles that stretch, the breath, and the bandhas. Understanding the joint positions enables you to determine the muscles that produce the posture. Engage the prime movers to sculpt the pose, and polish it with the synergists. Once you know the prime movers, you can identify the muscles that are stretching. Apply physiological techniques to lengthen these muscles and create mobility to deepen the pose.

Then there is the breath. In virtually every posture we can benefit from expanding the chest. Combine the accessory muscles of breathing with the action of the diaphragm to increase the volume of the thorax. This improves oxygenation of the blood and removes energetic blockages in the subtle body.

The bandhas are the finishing touch. Co-activate the muscle groups that produce the joint positions and you will create bandhas throughout the body. Then connect these peripheral locks to the core bandhas. This produces stability in the pose and accentuates the sensory imprint of the asana on the mind.

The Bandha Yoga Codex is a five-step process that teaches how to identify these elements and decode any pose. This is your guide to creating a road map for combining science and yoga. I use Natarajasana to illustrate the Codex on the following pages.

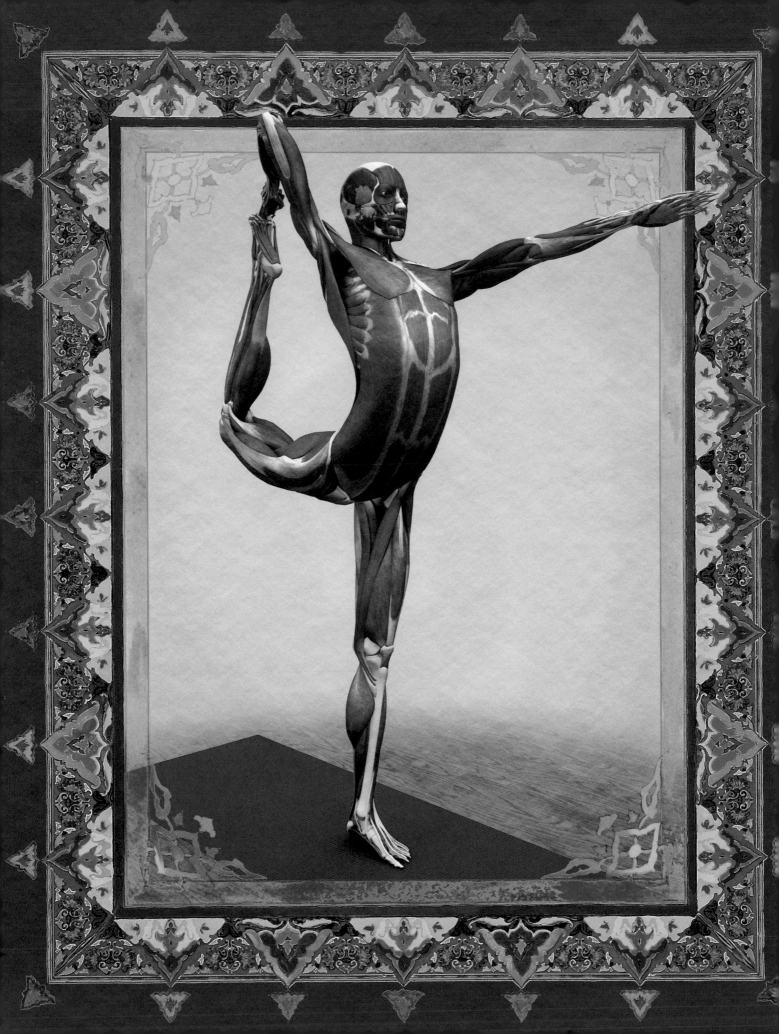

बन्ध योग

The Bandha Yoga Codex

— 1 —

Define the position of the joints in the pose.

— 2 —

Identify the prime mover muscles that act
on the joints to create the pose.
Contract these muscles to align and
stabilize the skeleton.

— 3 —

Identify the antagonist muscles
of the prime movers.
Stretch these muscles to create flexibility.

— 4 —

Expand the chest.

— 5 —

Create a Bandha.

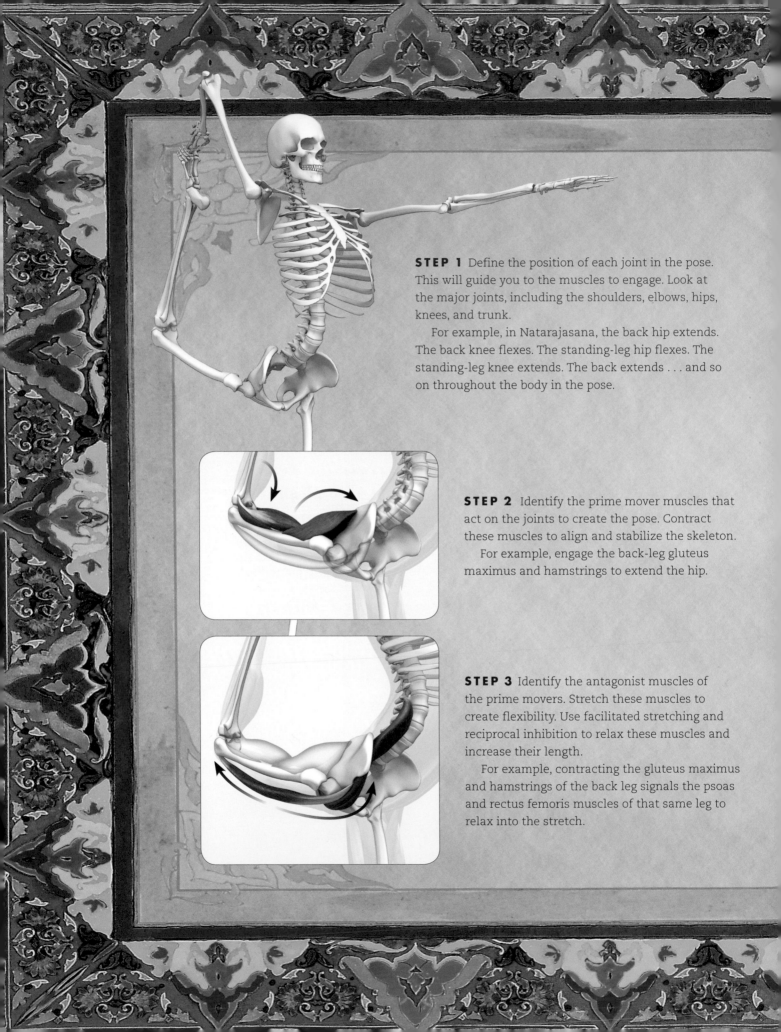

STEP 1 Define the position of each joint in the pose. This will guide you to the muscles to engage. Look at the major joints, including the shoulders, elbows, hips, knees, and trunk.

For example, in Natarajasana, the back hip extends. The back knee flexes. The standing-leg hip flexes. The standing-leg knee extends. The back extends . . . and so on throughout the body in the pose.

STEP 2 Identify the prime mover muscles that act on the joints to create the pose. Contract these muscles to align and stabilize the skeleton.

For example, engage the back-leg gluteus maximus and hamstrings to extend the hip.

STEP 3 Identify the antagonist muscles of the prime movers. Stretch these muscles to create flexibility. Use facilitated stretching and reciprocal inhibition to relax these muscles and increase their length.

For example, contracting the gluteus maximus and hamstrings of the back leg signals the psoas and rectus femoris muscles of that same leg to relax into the stretch.

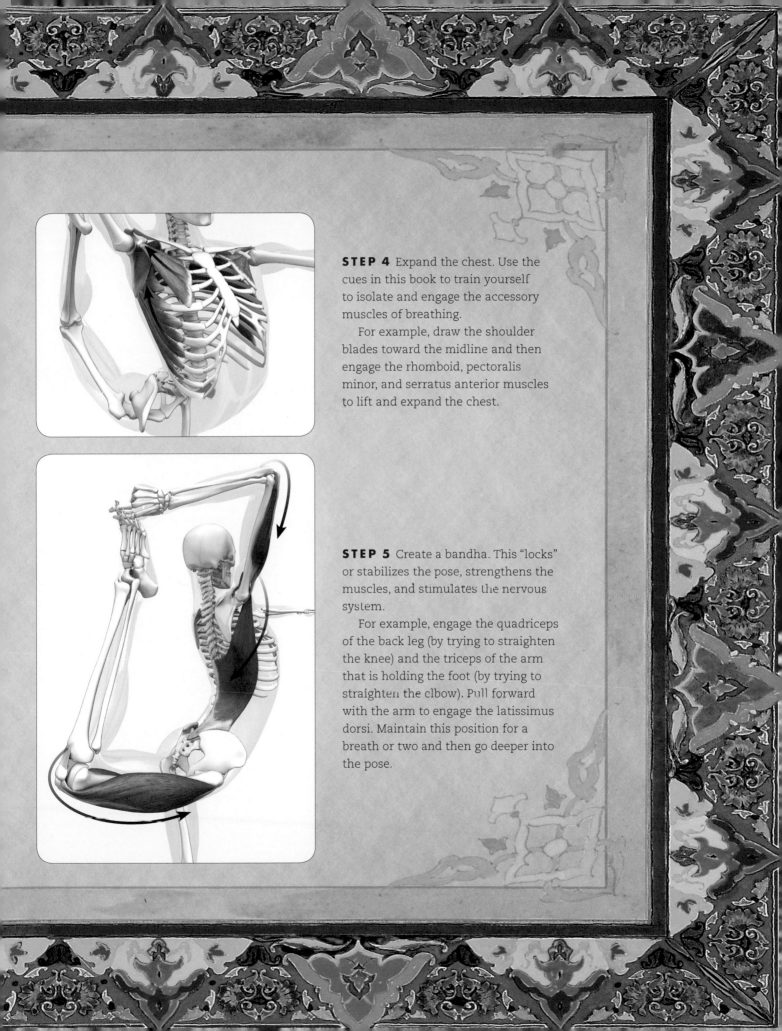

STEP 4 Expand the chest. Use the cues in this book to train yourself to isolate and engage the accessory muscles of breathing.

For example, draw the shoulder blades toward the midline and then engage the rhomboid, pectoralis minor, and serratus anterior muscles to lift and expand the chest.

STEP 5 Create a bandha. This "locks" or stabilizes the pose, strengthens the muscles, and stimulates the nervous system.

For example, engage the quadriceps of the back leg (by trying to straighten the knee) and the triceps of the arm that is holding the foot (by trying to straighten the elbow). Pull forward with the arm to engage the latissimus dorsi. Maintain this position for a breath or two and then go deeper into the pose.

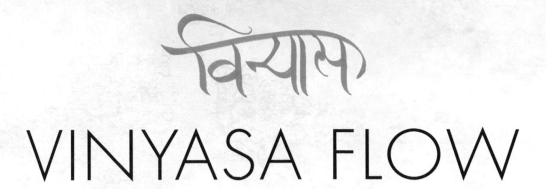

VINYASA FLOW

Vinyasa combines poses to flow, one into another, in sequence. Postures from the Sun Salutations form the foundation, which is repeated in successive rounds. Individual poses are then inserted into this foundation to create diversity within the flow. These asanas become the centerpiece of each round of Vinyasa. The flow sequence encircles the centerpiece pose and is the "home base" to which we return. Central to this practice is the coupling of breath and movement.

Vinyasa affects the body on many levels. It is an aerobic style of yoga that generates heat from muscle metabolism. Surface blood vessels then dilate to release this heat. This combines with sweating to maintain normal body temperature, producing a healthy glow to the skin and releasing toxins. Because you can sweat a great deal during practice, be sure to drink plenty of fluids to maintain hydration.

The repetitive nature of Vinyasa takes the joints through an increasingly greater range of motion, improving the circulation of synovial fluid and bringing nutrients to the articular cartilage. Working the muscles increases their metabolic rate, causing a slight rise in body temperature, which improves pliability in the ligaments and tendons. Alternately contracting and stretching the muscles during Vinyasa augments blood flow by compressing and expanding the veins. Cardiac output also increases. Rhythmic contraction and relaxation of the diaphragm during breathing massages the abdominal organs and improves

their function. Ujjayi breathing also produces a resonant sound that echoes throughout the physical body, connecting it to universal vibrational energies. Allow your breath to be the background soundtrack for your practice, like waves rolling onto a beach covered with smooth round stones. Breathing in this manner will eventually produce a self-sustaining rhythmic vibration. Combining breath and muscle work creates a symphony of movement and a resonance that will carry over into your daily life.

Vinyasa Flow can be used to warm up the body for other types of practice or can embody the practice itself. Think of Vinyasa Flow as a multi-layered system that combines breath work, muscle activation, and rhythmic movement. Transition smoothly from one pose to the next, and progressively refine each successive round as illustrated below. Begin by warming up the muscles that are the prime movers of the major joints. These are the muscles that create the general form of the pose. For example, in Downward Facing Dog, begin by engaging the quadriceps to straighten the knees and the triceps to extend the elbows. This stretches antagonist muscles, including the hamstrings and biceps. Consciously contracting the prime movers of the joints has the additional physiological effect of relaxing their antagonist muscles through reciprocal inhibition. As your practice session progresses, incorporate other muscles to refine the poses. The following pages illustrate this concept.

VINYASA: UJJAYI BREATHING

During the first few cycles of Vinyasa practice, focus on your breath. Engaging the respiratory muscles moves air in and out of the lungs, oxygenating the blood and removing carbon dioxide. The alveoli in the lungs are microscopic sac-like structures that have a thin membrane separating air from the blood in the capillaries. This is where gas exchange takes place. These alveoli are elastic in nature, expanding like a balloon on inhalation and then passively recoiling back down to size on exhalation. Oxygenated blood is transported by the circulatory system from the lungs to the tissues of the body, where it is consumed for metabolism. Carbon dioxide is produced in the tissues as a by-product of metabolism and is transported to the lungs for release into the air.

The main muscle of respiration is the diaphragm. It is a thin, dome-shaped muscle that separates the chest cavity from the abdomen. Contracting the diaphragm during inhalation causes the dome to flatten out. This increases the volume of the chest cavity and draws air into the lungs via the trachea and bronchi. The diaphragm functions unconsciously, so that it contracts without you thinking about it. You can also contract it consciously, which is what happens if you intentionally breathe faster or more deeply. Exhalation is a passive process that occurs as a result of the elastic recoil of the chest wall and the sac-like alveoli. As you exhale, the diaphragm relaxes back into its dome shape, decreasing the volume of the chest.

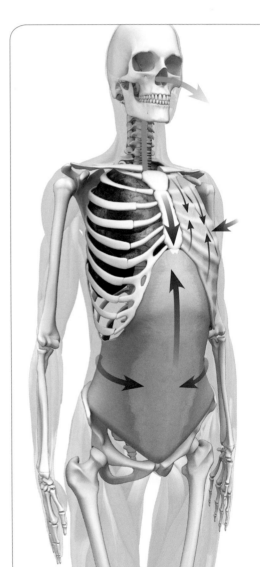

FIGURE 1 Make exhalation a more active process when practicing Vinyasa Flow. Do this by gently engaging the abdominal muscles, activating the rectus and transversus abdominis. Slightly squeeze the chest as well to contract the muscles that connect one rib to another: the internal intercostals.

Activating the transversus abdominis increases intra-abdominal pressure. This increased pressure causes the abdominal organs to be lifted up against the diaphragm, aiding to empty the lungs. Contracting the internal intercostals brings the ribs closer together, thus decreasing the volume of the thorax (the chest) during exhalation.

Bear in mind that the lungs are never completely empty. There is always what is called the "residual volume" that remains in the non-compressible elements of the respiratory system—the bronchi and trachea. Contracting the abdominal and intercostal muscles expels some of the air remaining in the elastic, sac-like structures of the lungs where gas exchange takes place. Make exhalation an active process during Vinyasa to decrease this residual volume. This aids to remove more of the carbon dioxide that is produced during metabolism.

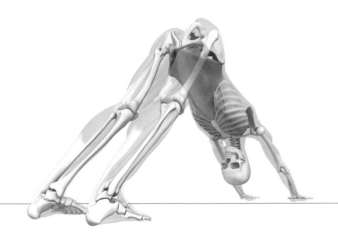

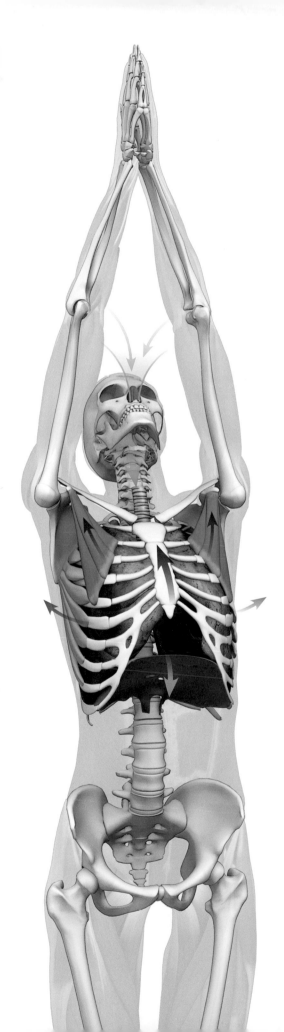

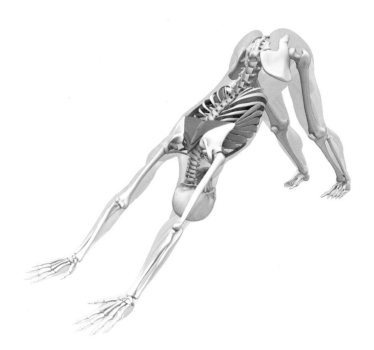

FIGURE 2 Inhalation is, for the most part, driven by the diaphragm. The phrenic nerve controls this muscle, which functions both consciously and unconsciously. The diaphragm will do its work automatically, but you can direct the frequency and depth of each inhalation.

The brain can recruit the accessory muscles of breathing to increase ventilation when the body needs more oxygen. Watch a sprinter at the end of a race, and you will see that they are engaging muscles in the neck, back, chest, and abdomen to increase lung volume. This happens automatically when more oxygen is needed and more carbon dioxide must be expelled.

You can augment the depth of inhalation during Vinyasa by training yourself to contract certain of the accessory muscles of breathing. I primarily use a combination of the rhomboids, pectoralis minor, and serratus anterior. Begin by engaging the rhomboids to draw the shoulder blades toward the midline. This opens the chest forward. Fix the shoulder blades in place, and then expand the chest upward and outward by activating the pectoralis minor and serratus anterior muscles. A cue for isolating the pectoralis minor is to attempt to roll the shoulders forward; at the same time, activate the rhomboids to prevent the shoulders from moving. As a result, the contractile force of the pectoralis minor is transmitted to its origin on the ribcage, lifting it. To engage the serratus anterior, imagine pushing outwards against a doorway with the hands. Note how this expands the chest.

The serratus anterior and pectoralis minor muscles can be difficult to access at first. Therefore, I recommend simply "going through the motions" at the beginning of your practice a few times—like making a rough sketch. Then leave it. For the rest of your practice simply breathe deeply. In the time between sessions, your unconscious brain will honor your effort and form circuitry to more efficiently activate the accessory muscles of breathing at your command. Don't try too hard and don't give up.

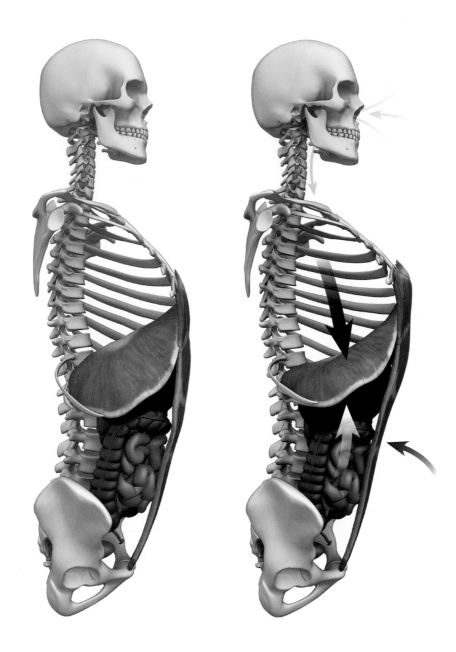

FIGURE 3 Just as squeezing the abdomen exerts an upwardly directed pressure on the diaphragm, so does the rhythmic contraction of the diaphragm flatten to compress and massage the abdominal organs. Then, as the diaphragm relaxes and returns to its dome shape, the abdominal organs are drawn upward. This creates a "pumping" type of action on the blood-filled sinusoids of the liver and spleen, improving circulation through these organs and detoxifying the blood. The lymphatics that surround the intestines are massaged, stimulating the immune system. The rhythmic pumping action of yogic breathing on the stomach and intestines also improves digestion and elimination.

Gently activating the abdominal muscles during Vinyasa tones them, while at the same time raising the intra-abdominal pressure. This increased pressure creates a resistance for the diaphragm to contract against as it flattens, exercising and strengthening it.

FIGURE 4 The glottis surrounds and includes the opening between the pharynx and trachea (windpipe). You can decrease the size of this opening by contracting the muscles of the glottis. Decreasing the size of this aperture creates turbulent airflow, producing the characteristic sound of ujjayi breathing. This sound resonates through the chest, which functions like a speaker box. The rhythmic sound of ujjayi (sometimes called "ocean breath") is reminiscent of waves on the beach.

Air is warmed as it passes over the blood-rich mucosa that lines the nasal sinuses and pharynx. Creating turbulence within the glottis increases the time that the air is in contact with this mucosal lining, warming it further. This forms part of the basis for pranayama.

Finally, there is a biomechanical benefit to working with ujjayi breathing in yoga. Narrowing the opening of the glottis creates a resistance to airflow into the lungs. Thus the diaphragm has to work a little bit harder to draw the air in, giving this muscle a light workout. Strengthening the diaphragm during yogic breathing has benefits that carry over into your daily life, as breathing feels lighter and easier.

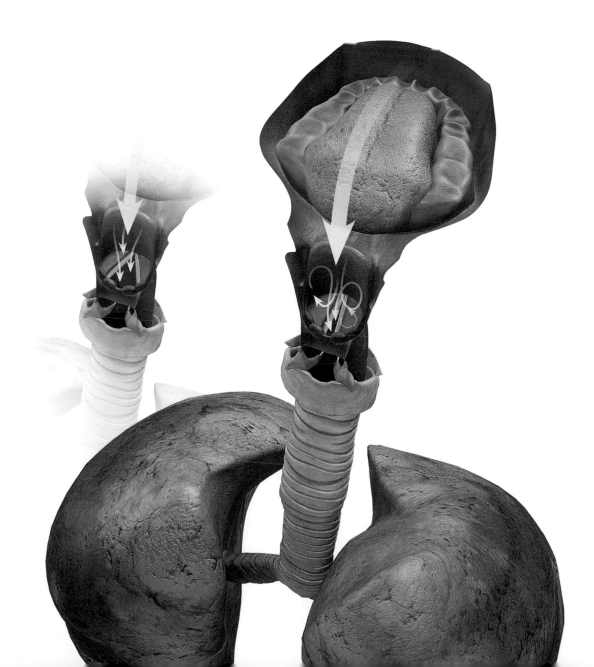

VINYASA: FOUNDATION POSES
TADASANA (MOUNTAIN POSE)

The following pages illustrate muscles that can be activated in successive rounds of Vinyasa Flow. Each round deepens the postures as the body warms up. Each suggested muscle group, in turn, refines the poses. The figures below are numbered for consecutive rounds of the series.

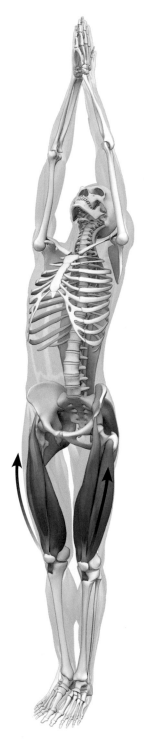

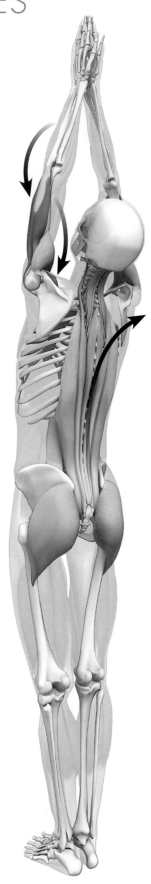

◀ **FIGURE 1** Begin by contracting the quadriceps. The cue for this is to lift the kneecaps and straighten the knees.

▶ **FIGURE 2** Next, engage the gluteus maximus, erector spinae, and quadratus lumborum to lift and slightly arch the back. Raise the arms by activating the anterior deltoids. You can feel these muscles contract at the fronts of the shoulders during this movement. Straighten the elbows by engaging the triceps. The long head of the triceps also rotates the scapula. Activating this muscle enables you to lift the arms higher.

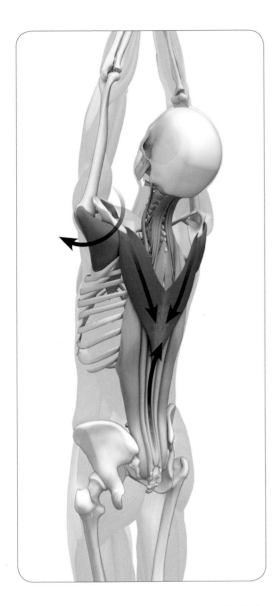

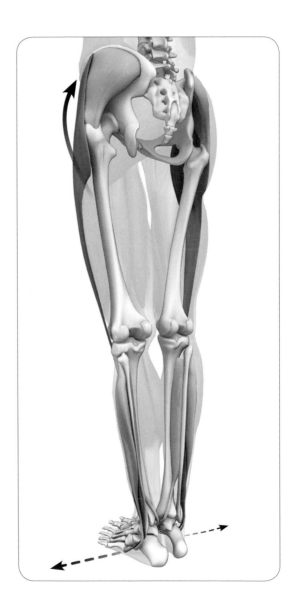

▼ **FIGURE 4** Press the balls of the feet into the mat by contracting the peroneus longus and brevis muscles on the outsides of the lower legs. Then attempt to draw the soles of the feet apart. They will not move because the mat constrains them, but this cue for abducting the feet will activate the tensor fascia lata and gluteus medius at the sides of the hips. These muscles, which also internally rotate the thighs, will turn the femurs inward and bring the kneecaps to face forward.

▲ **FIGURE 3** Contract the lower third of the trapezius to draw the shoulders away from the ears and free the neck. Use the image to help you visualize this muscle. Externally rotate the shoulders by engaging the infraspinatus and teres minor muscles of the rotator cuff.

VINYASA: FOUNDATION POSES
UTTANASANA (INTENSE FORWARD-BENDING POSE)

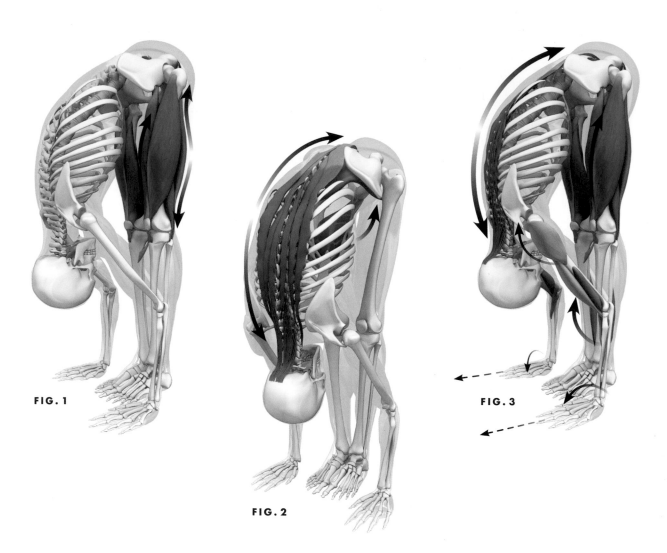

FIG. 1

FIG. 2

FIG. 3

FIGURE 1 Activate the quadriceps as you bend forward into Uttanasana. Train yourself to gradually increase the force of this muscle contracting as you go into the pose. This acts to straighten the knees, stretching the hamstrings. Engaging the quadriceps also produces reciprocal inhibition of the hamstrings, helping them to relax into the stretch.

FIGURE 2 In the next round, engage the hip flexors (the psoas and its synergists) and the abdominals to flex the hips and bend the trunk forward. Attempt to squeeze the torso against the thighs to contract the psoas. Activating these muscles signals the gluteus maximus, erector spinae, and quadratus lumborum to relax into the stretch.

FIGURE 3 Plant the hands firmly onto the mat by pressing down the mounds at the base of the index fingers. Attempt to drag the hands forward away from the feet by contracting the anterior deltoids and biceps. Because the hands are fixed and won't move, these muscles act to flex the torso further into the pose. As you deepen the asana, create a bandha by engaging the quadriceps. This signals the hamstrings to relax into the stretch due to reciprocal inhibition.

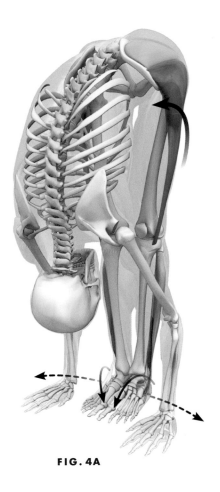

FIG. 4A

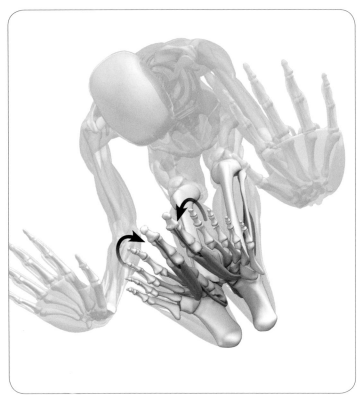

FIG. 4B

FIGURE 4A For this round, press the balls of the feet into the mat by engaging the peronei at the sides of the lower legs. Then attempt to drag the feet apart, thereby engaging the tensor fascia lata and gluteus medius. This cue internally rotates the thighs, bringing the kneecaps to face forward.

FIGURE 4B The pelvis tends to drift back in this pose. Counter this by pressing the fleshy part of the big toes into the mat. This engages the big toe flexors. Note how this works to bring the pelvis forward, aligning it over the ankles.

VINYASA: FOUNDATION POSES
CHATURANGA DANDASANA (FOUR-LIMB STAFF POSE)

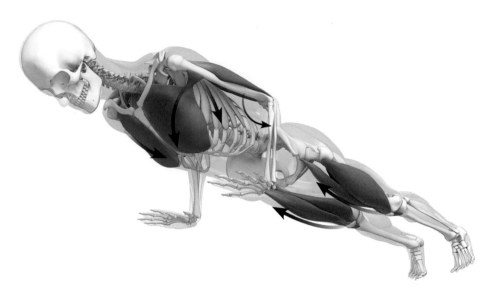

▲ **FIGURE 1** Typically, we jump or step back into Chaturanga Dandasana from Uttanasana. Relax when lowering, and then at the last moment, activate the pectoralis major to hold the upper body off the floor. A cue for accessing this muscle is to attempt to draw the elbows toward one another. At the same time, engage the serratus anterior to stabilize the scapulae (the shoulder blades) and prevent them from "winging" upward off the back. Use the image to visualize this muscle contracting. Support the elbows by activating the triceps. This prevents the elbows from bending more than ninety degrees and maintains the forearms at a right angle to the floor. Engage the quadriceps to straighten the knees. The cue for this is to lift and draw the kneecaps toward the pelvis.

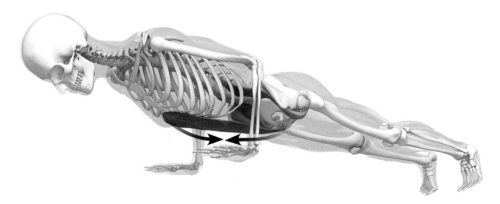

▲ **FIGURE 2** There can be a tendency for the body to sag a bit when lowering into Chaturanga Dandasana. Anticipate this and prepare to counteract it. Relax the body when jumping back, and then, before the body sags, engage the rectus abdominis and psoas muscles to support the midsection and pelvis and maintain the body as a plank (the common name for this pose).

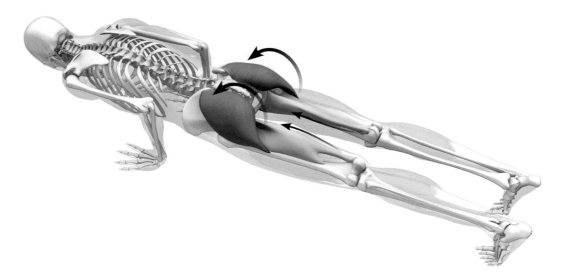

▲ **FIGURE 3** Balance the hip-flexing action of the psoas by engaging the main hip extensor, the gluteus maximus. This produces opposing forces across the pelvis, thereby creating a bandha. Synergize the gluteus maximus by activating the adductor magnus, which in addition to drawing the legs together, also extends the hips. The cue for contracting this muscle is to attempt to gently squeeze the legs towards one another.

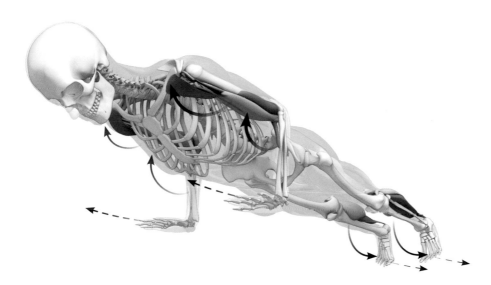

▲ **FIGURE 4** Once you are warmed up from doing a few rounds of Vinyasa, attempt to "scrub" the hands forward while at the same time trying to press the feet backwards (as if you were pushing out of a runner's starting blocks). Press the mounds of the index fingers into the mat to engage the pronators teres and quadratus of the forearms. Then attempt to bend the elbows and scrub the hands forward to activate the biceps, brachialis, and anterior deltoid muscles. The elbows won't actually bend and the hands won't move, but the force of contracting these muscles stabilizes the shoulders and upper extremities. Pressing off with the feet activates the gastrocnemius and soleus muscles of the calves, stabilizing the ankles. The net effect of this action—scrubbing forward with the hands while pressing off with the feet— is the creation of a bandha throughout the body that helps to stabilize the pose.

VINYASA: FOUNDATION POSES
URDHVA MUKHA SVANASANA (UPWARD FACING DOG POSE)

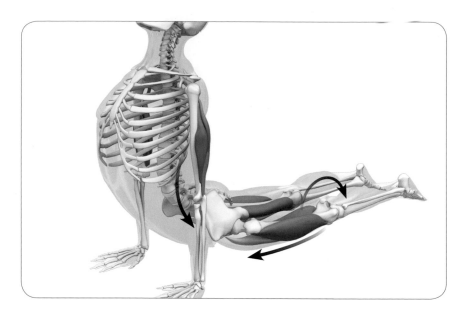

▲ **FIGURE 1** Take the general form of Upward Facing Dog Pose by straightening the elbows and extending the knees. Do this by contracting the triceps and quadriceps.

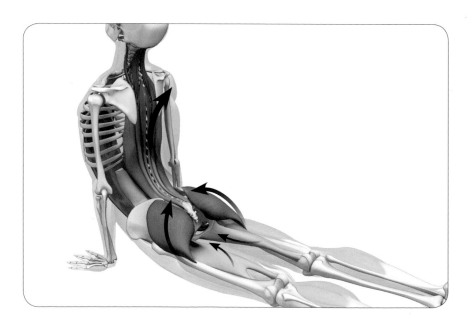

▲ **FIGURE 2** On the next round, firm the buttocks to engage the gluteus maximus. This extends the hips and, at the same time, signals the hip flexors (the psoas and its synergists) to relax through reciprocal inhibition. Add to this the adductor magnus, a synergist of the gluteus maximus that also extends the hips. To activate this muscle, gently draw the legs together.

Then, move up the back and into the trunk to contract the spine extensors, including the erector spinae and quadratus lumborum. Engaging these muscles produces reciprocal inhibition of the abdominals at the front of the torso, relaxing them into the stretch.

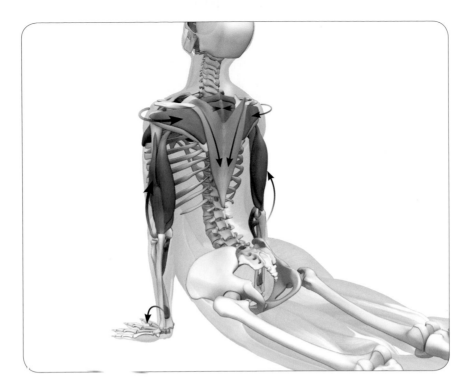

▲ **FIGURE 3** Now focus on the arms and shoulders. Press the mounds at the base of the index fingers into the mat, engaging the pronators teres and quadratus. Move up the arms to the triceps, contracting them to straighten the elbows. Then externally rotate the shoulders by activating the infraspinatus and teres minor muscles of the rotator cuff. Working your way up the arms in this fashion produces a combination of opposing actions—internally rotating the forearms and externally rotating the shoulders. This creates a helical bandha in the arms, stabilizing them.

Complete the round by engaging the rhomboids and lower third of the trapezius to draw the shoulder blades together and down the back. This opens the chest and frees the neck.

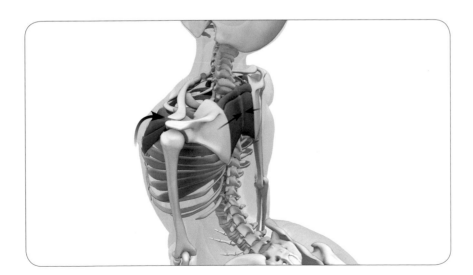

▲ **FIGURE 4** Finally, use the accessory muscles of breathing to expand the ribcage. Hold the shoulder blades (the scapulae) in place with the rhomboids. Then lift the ribcage upward with the pectoralis minor, and expand the chest outward with the serratus anterior. Inhale deeply as you go into Upward Facing Dog. These muscles help you to do this.

VINYASA: FOUNDATION POSES
ADHO MUKHA SVANASANA (DOWNWARD FACING DOG POSE)

Relax and take five breaths in Dog Pose. Work through the body with each successive breath.

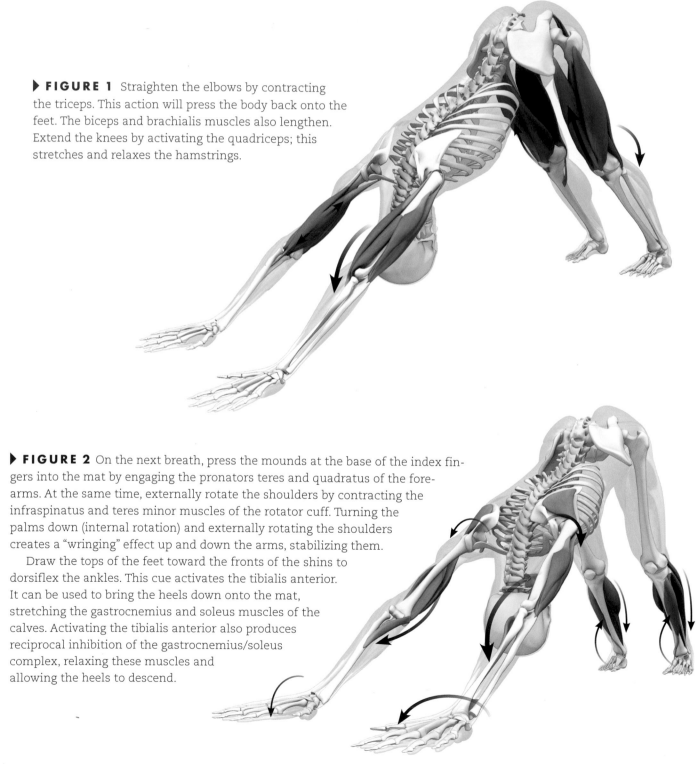

▶ **FIGURE 1** Straighten the elbows by contracting the triceps. This action will press the body back onto the feet. The biceps and brachialis muscles also lengthen. Extend the knees by activating the quadriceps; this stretches and relaxes the hamstrings.

▶ **FIGURE 2** On the next breath, press the mounds at the base of the index fingers into the mat by engaging the pronators teres and quadratus of the forearms. At the same time, externally rotate the shoulders by contracting the infraspinatus and teres minor muscles of the rotator cuff. Turning the palms down (internal rotation) and externally rotating the shoulders creates a "wringing" effect up and down the arms, stabilizing them.

Draw the tops of the feet toward the fronts of the shins to dorsiflex the ankles. This cue activates the tibialis anterior. It can be used to bring the heels down onto the mat, stretching the gastrocnemius and soleus muscles of the calves. Activating the tibialis anterior also produces reciprocal inhibition of the gastrocnemius/soleus complex, relaxing these muscles and allowing the heels to descend.

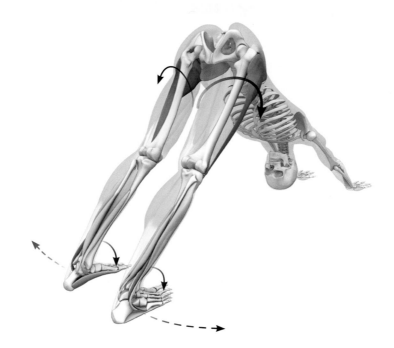

▲ **FIGURE 3** Next, press the balls of the feet into the mat to engage the peroneus longus and brevis muscles at the sides of the lower legs. Then attempt to drag the feet out to the side, away from one another. The feet remain constrained on the mat, but this cue engages the abductor muscles at the sides of the hips—the gluteus medius and tensor fascia lata. These muscles originate from the iliac crests. Contracting them in this way pulls on the iliac crests, freeing the sacroiliac joints so that the sacrum can tilt forward—a movement known as nutation. Note how this deepens your pose. The main hip abductors also internally rotate the thighs. As a result, engaging them turns the femurs in slightly, bringing the kneecaps to face forward.

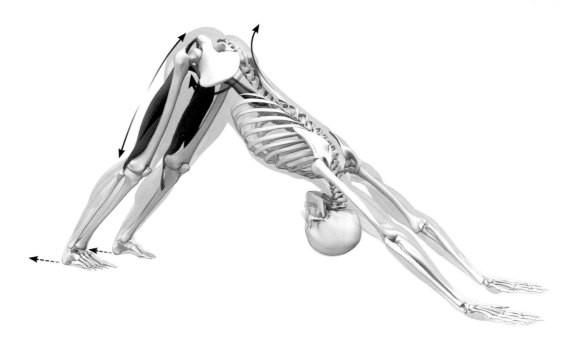

▲ **FIGURE 4** Complete Downward Facing Dog Pose by contracting the quadratus lumborum and erector spinae muscles to extend the lumbar spine and the psoas to flex the hips. These muscles also tilt the pelvis forward into anteversion. Arching the lower back, tilting the pelvis forward, and flexing the hips draws the origin of the hamstrings, the ischial tuberosities or sitting bones, upward. This action stretches the hamstrings. At the same time, activate the quadriceps to produce reciprocal inhibition of the hamstrings, relaxing them into the final part of the pose.

VINYASA: FOUNDATION POSES
JUMPING THROUGH

The foundational Vinyasa sequence can be varied to accommodate poses that are seated or supine, such as forward bends or backbends. In this variation, instead of returning to Tadasana, we jump or step through the arms into Dandasana, or Staff Pose. This requires some training of the muscles of the upper body, trunk, and pelvis. You can also use blocks to gain extra height for lifting the body.

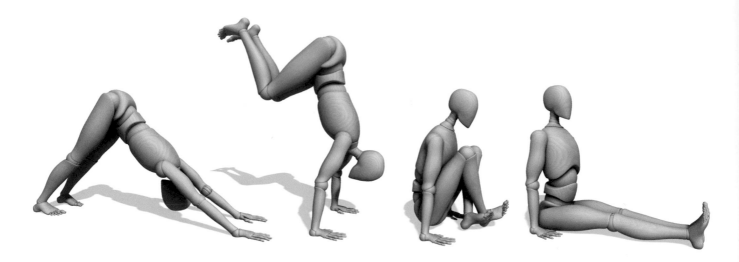

▲ **FIGURE 1** This image illustrates the entire sequence. Jump forward from Dog Pose, lifting the legs and slightly arching the back by contracting the hip and back extensors—the gluteus maximus and quadratus lumborum. This is a key to bringing the trunk over the shoulders. These muscles help to produce the momentum that is critical for this technique. Then, once the trunk and pelvis are lifted, fold the hips into flexion to bring the feet between the arms, as shown.

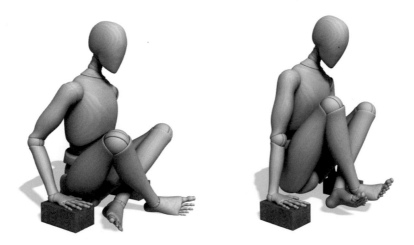

▲ **FIGURE 2** Use blocks to gain height and to get a feeling for lifting the body with the arms. In the beginning, you may need to keep the feet on the floor. This is fine, as it will build the strength necessary to eventually lift the weight of the legs as well.

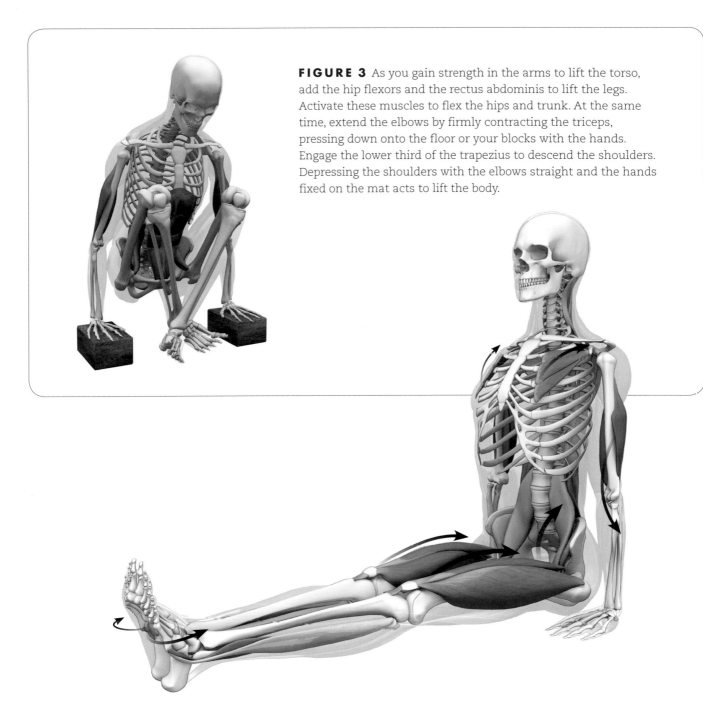

FIGURE 3 As you gain strength in the arms to lift the torso, add the hip flexors and the rectus abdominis to lift the legs. Activate these muscles to flex the hips and trunk. At the same time, extend the elbows by firmly contracting the triceps, pressing down onto the floor or your blocks with the hands. Engage the lower third of the trapezius to descend the shoulders. Depressing the shoulders with the elbows straight and the hands fixed on the mat acts to lift the body.

FIGURE 4 Jump or step through into Dandasana. Once in the pose, make it active by engaging the quadriceps to straighten the knees. The feet tend to "sickle" or turn inward. Counter this by opening the soles of the feet outward, everting the ankles slightly. This cue contracts the peronei on the sides of the lower legs. Then activate the toe extensors by drawing the toes toward the trunk. These actions—everting the ankles and extending the toes—open the soles of the feet. Balance this by engaging the tibialis posterior muscles to stabilize the bones of the lower legs. This inverts the ankles and dynamizes the arches.

Move up the body into the hips, flexing them by engaging the psoas. The psoas also acts synergistically with the quadratus lumborum to lift and create a slight arch in the lower back. Press down with the hands by extending the elbows, using the triceps. Contract the forearm pronators to press the index finger sides of the hands into the mat, and then spread the weight evenly across the palms.

Finally, on your inhalation, engage the rhomboids to draw the shoulder blades toward the midline, opening the chest forward. Then lift and expand the ribcage by contracting the pectoralis minor and serratus anterior.

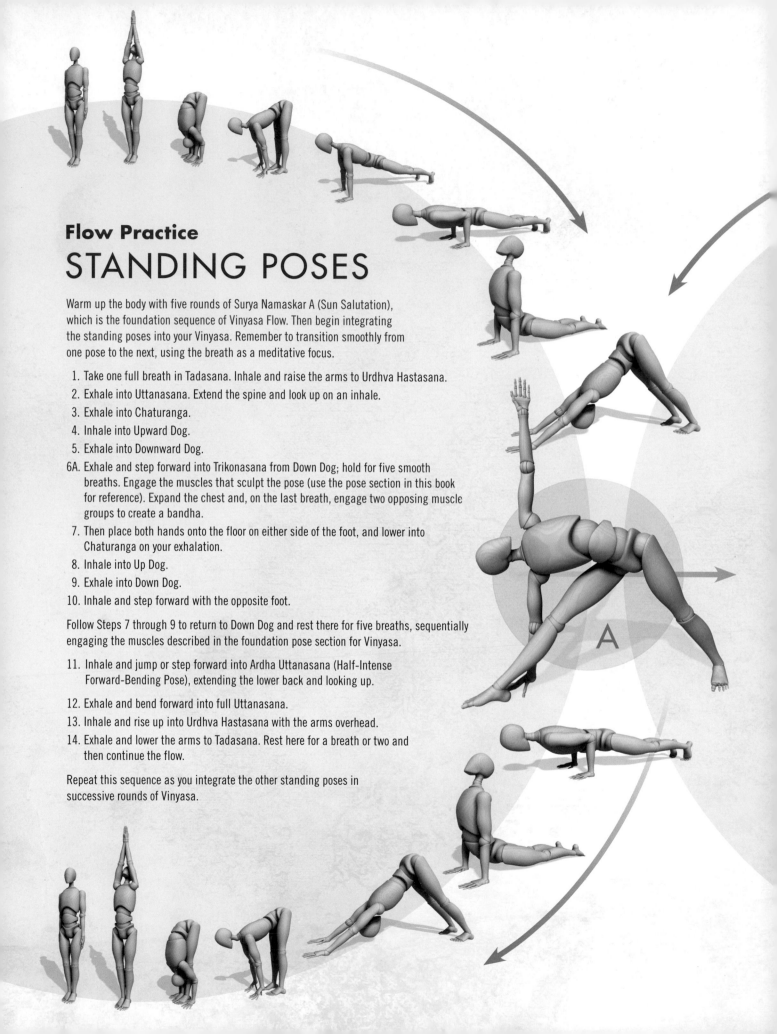

Flow Practice
STANDING POSES

Warm up the body with five rounds of Surya Namaskar A (Sun Salutation), which is the foundation sequence of Vinyasa Flow. Then begin integrating the standing poses into your Vinyasa. Remember to transition smoothly from one pose to the next, using the breath as a meditative focus.

1. Take one full breath in Tadasana. Inhale and raise the arms to Urdhva Hastasana.
2. Exhale into Uttanasana. Extend the spine and look up on an inhale.
3. Exhale into Chaturanga.
4. Inhale into Upward Dog.
5. Exhale into Downward Dog.
6A. Exhale and step forward into Trikonasana from Down Dog; hold for five smooth breaths. Engage the muscles that sculpt the pose (use the pose section in this book for reference). Expand the chest and, on the last breath, engage two opposing muscle groups to create a bandha.
7. Then place both hands onto the floor on either side of the foot, and lower into Chaturanga on your exhalation.
8. Inhale into Up Dog.
9. Exhale into Down Dog.
10. Inhale and step forward with the opposite foot.

Follow Steps 7 through 9 to return to Down Dog and rest there for five breaths, sequentially engaging the muscles described in the foundation pose section for Vinyasa.

11. Inhale and jump or step forward into Ardha Uttanasana (Half-Intense Forward-Bending Pose), extending the lower back and looking up.

12. Exhale and bend forward into full Uttanasana.
13. Inhale and rise up into Urdhva Hastasana with the arms overhead.
14. Exhale and lower the arms to Tadasana. Rest here for a breath or two and then continue the flow.

Repeat this sequence as you integrate the other standing poses in successive rounds of Vinyasa.

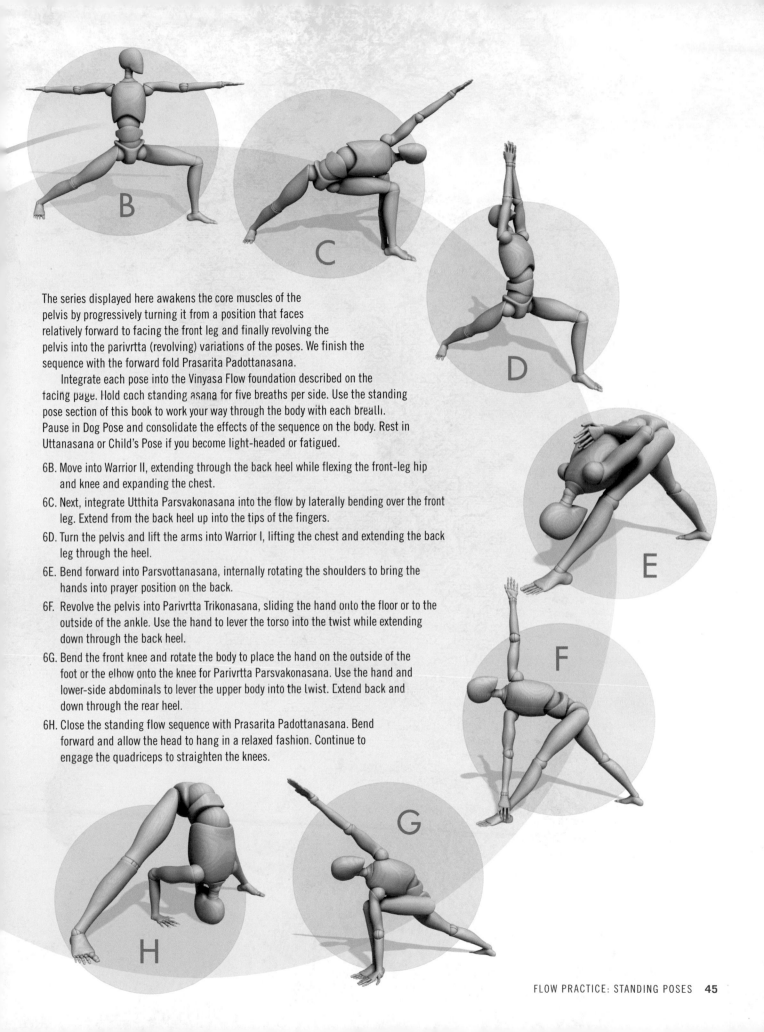

The series displayed here awakens the core muscles of the pelvis by progressively turning it from a position that faces relatively forward to facing the front leg and finally revolving the pelvis into the parivrtta (revolving) variations of the poses. We finish the sequence with the forward fold Prasarita Padottanasana.

Integrate each pose into the Vinyasa Flow foundation described on the facing page. Hold each standing asana for five breaths per side. Use the standing pose section of this book to work your way through the body with each breath. Pause in Dog Pose and consolidate the effects of the sequence on the body. Rest in Uttanasana or Child's Pose if you become light-headed or fatigued.

6B. Move into Warrior II, extending through the back heel while flexing the front-leg hip and knee and expanding the chest.

6C. Next, integrate Utthita Parsvakonasana into the flow by laterally bending over the front leg. Extend from the back heel up into the tips of the fingers.

6D. Turn the pelvis and lift the arms into Warrior I, lifting the chest and extending the back leg through the heel.

6E. Bend forward into Parsvottanasana, internally rotating the shoulders to bring the hands into prayer position on the back.

6F. Revolve the pelvis into Parivrtta Trikonasana, sliding the hand onto the floor or to the outside of the ankle. Use the hand to lever the torso into the twist while extending down through the back heel.

6G. Bend the front knee and rotate the body to place the hand on the outside of the foot or the elbow onto the knee for Parivrtta Parsvakonasana. Use the hand and lower-side abdominals to lever the upper body into the twist. Extend back and down through the rear heel.

6H. Close the standing flow sequence with Prasarita Padottanasana. Bend forward and allow the head to hang in a relaxed fashion. Continue to engage the quadriceps to straighten the knees.

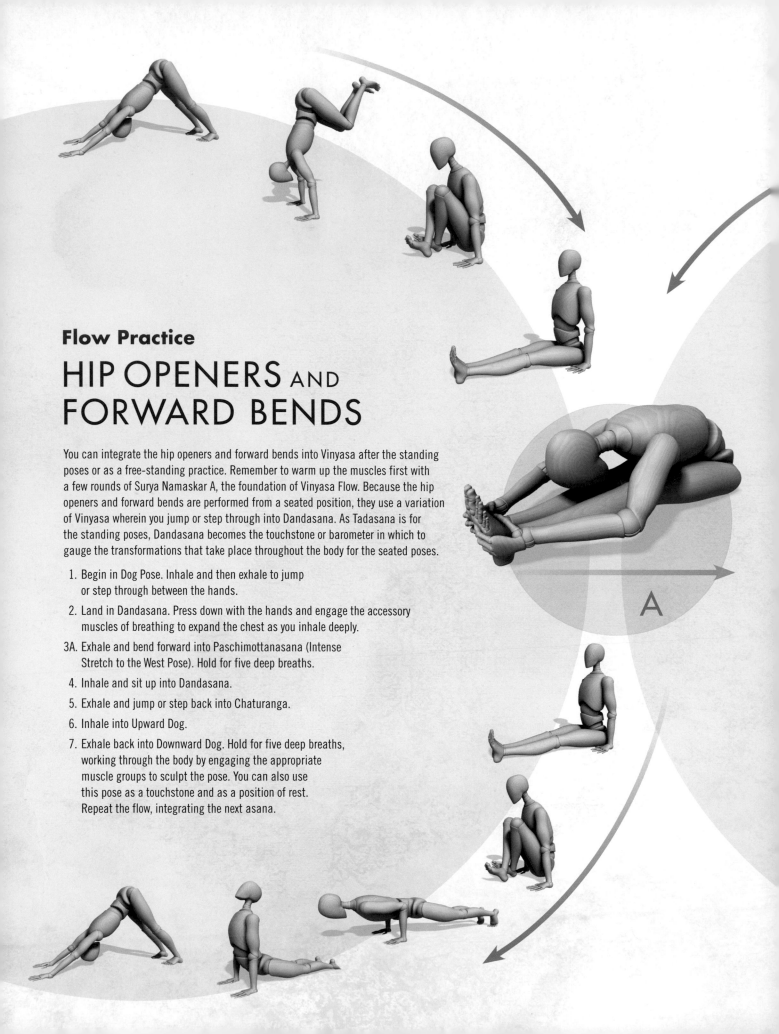

Flow Practice
HIP OPENERS AND FORWARD BENDS

You can integrate the hip openers and forward bends into Vinyasa after the standing poses or as a free-standing practice. Remember to warm up the muscles first with a few rounds of Surya Namaskar A, the foundation of Vinyasa Flow. Because the hip openers and forward bends are performed from a seated position, they use a variation of Vinyasa wherein you jump or step through into Dandasana. As Tadasana is for the standing poses, Dandasana becomes the touchstone or barometer in which to gauge the transformations that take place throughout the body for the seated poses.

1. Begin in Dog Pose. Inhale and then exhale to jump or step through between the hands.

2. Land in Dandasana. Press down with the hands and engage the accessory muscles of breathing to expand the chest as you inhale deeply.

3A. Exhale and bend forward into Paschimottanasana (Intense Stretch to the West Pose). Hold for five deep breaths.

4. Inhale and sit up into Dandasana.

5. Exhale and jump or step back into Chaturanga.

6. Inhale into Upward Dog.

7. Exhale back into Downward Dog. Hold for five deep breaths, working through the body by engaging the appropriate muscle groups to sculpt the pose. You can also use this pose as a touchstone and as a position of rest. Repeat the flow, integrating the next asana.

A

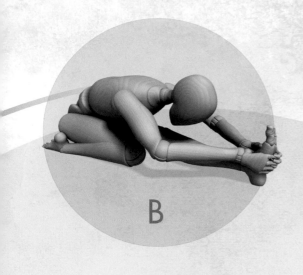

B

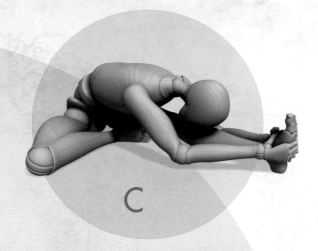

C

In this series, we begin with forward bends and close with hip openers. Refer to Mat Companion 2 for details on the muscles you engage and stretch in these poses. Integrate the postures into the flow, holding each for five breaths, as described for Paschimottanasana on the facing page.

3B. Take Triang Mukhaikapada Paschimottanasana (Three Limbs Face One Foot Pose), bending one knee and straightening the other. This is an asymmetrical pose in which the tendency is to lean to the straight-leg side. Balance this by engaging the muscles that push and draw you towards the bent-knee side. Repeat on the other side.

3C. Flex, abduct, and externally rotate the hip on one side, bending the knee to form Janu Sirsasana (Head-to-Knee Pose). Extend the other knee and reach forward to grasp the foot.

3D. Flex, abduct, and externally rotate both hips into Baddha Konasana (Bound Angle Pose). Squeeze the lower legs against the thighs to flex the knees.

3E. Spread the legs apart and reach forward to grasp the feet to take Upavistha Konasana (Wide-Angle Seated Forward Bend Pose).

3F. Finish with Kurmasana (Tortoise Pose), placing the arms under the knees or thighs and flexing the trunk forward.

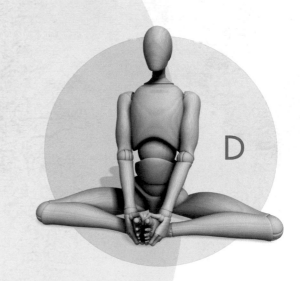

D

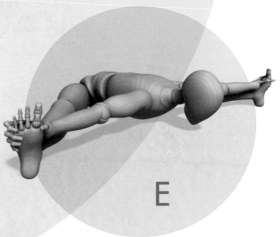

E

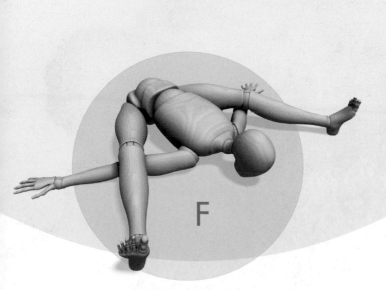

F

FLOW PRACTICE: HIP OPENERS AND FORWARD BENDS **47**

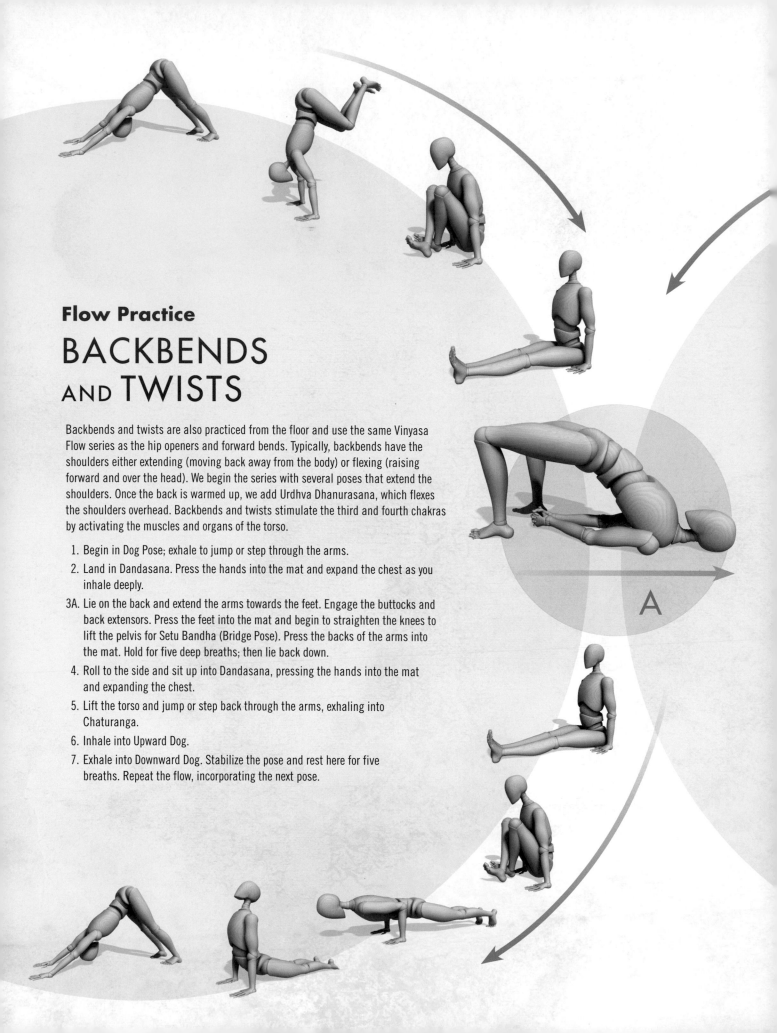

Flow Practice
BACKBENDS
AND TWISTS

Backbends and twists are also practiced from the floor and use the same Vinyasa Flow series as the hip openers and forward bends. Typically, backbends have the shoulders either extending (moving back away from the body) or flexing (raising forward and over the head). We begin the series with several poses that extend the shoulders. Once the back is warmed up, we add Urdhva Dhanurasana, which flexes the shoulders overhead. Backbends and twists stimulate the third and fourth chakras by activating the muscles and organs of the torso.

1. Begin in Dog Pose; exhale to jump or step through the arms.

2. Land in Dandasana. Press the hands into the mat and expand the chest as you inhale deeply.

3A. Lie on the back and extend the arms towards the feet. Engage the buttocks and back extensors. Press the feet into the mat and begin to straighten the knees to lift the pelvis for Setu Bandha (Bridge Pose). Press the backs of the arms into the mat. Hold for five deep breaths; then lie back down.

4. Roll to the side and sit up into Dandasana, pressing the hands into the mat and expanding the chest.

5. Lift the torso and jump or step back through the arms, exhaling into Chaturanga.

6. Inhale into Upward Dog.

7. Exhale into Downward Dog. Stabilize the pose and rest here for five breaths. Repeat the flow, incorporating the next pose.

A

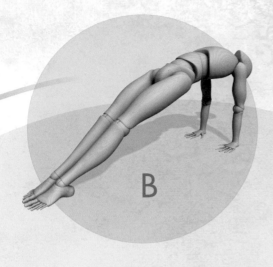

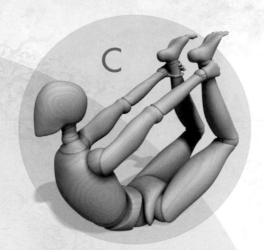

3B. Next, integrate Purvottanasana (Inclined Plane Pose) into the flow. Press the hands into the mat and firmly extend the elbows. At the same time, straighten the knees and press the soles of the feet into the floor.

3C. Turn onto the stomach and grasp the ankles for Dhanurasana (Bow Pose). Create a bandha by attempting to straighten the knees while resisting by trying to bend the elbows.

3D. Push up into Urdhva Dhanurasana (Upward Facing Bow Pose). Note how the shoulders are now flexing overhead (as opposed to extending in the previous poses). Combine the actions of the shoulders and hips and the elbows and knees to balance the body weight over the hands and feet.

3E. Backbends engage the extensor muscles of the back. Twists balance some of this contraction by stretching the spinal rotators. Start with a seated twist, using the arms to turn the body. Engage the core abdominal muscles to stabilize the torso.

3F. Move into a deeper twist with Marichyasana III (Great Sage Pose).

Integrate these twists into the flow, as shown on the previous page.

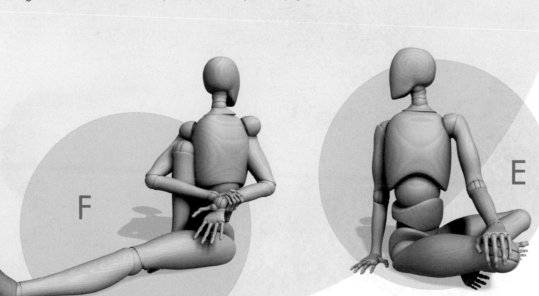

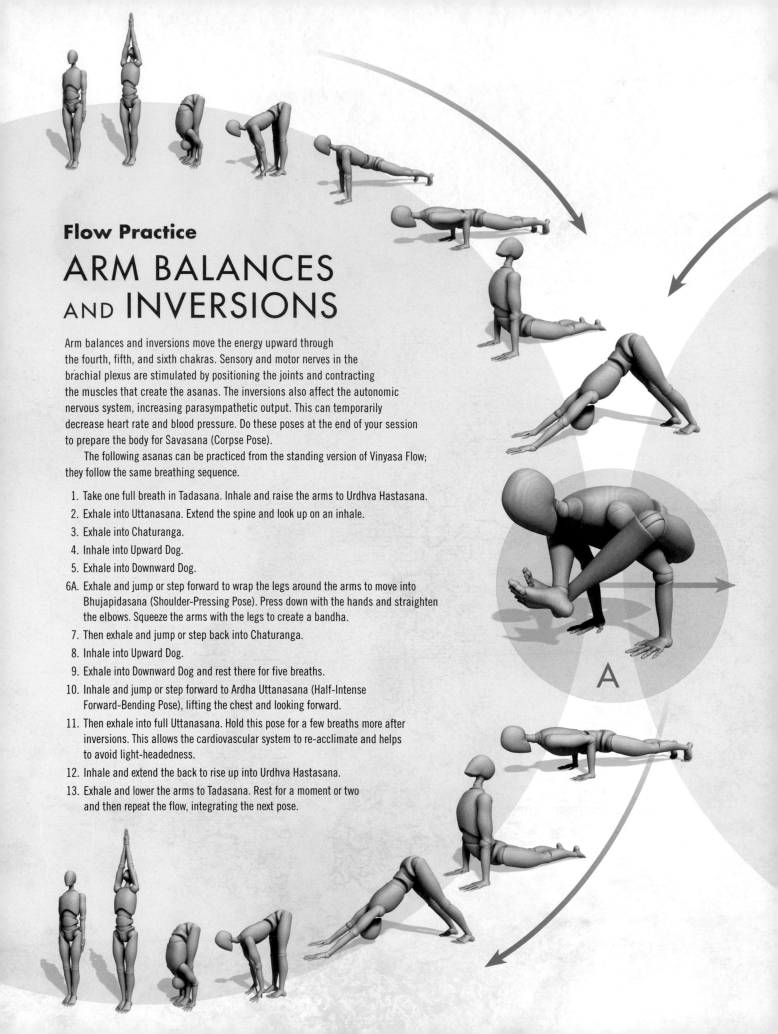

Flow Practice

ARM BALANCES AND INVERSIONS

Arm balances and inversions move the energy upward through the fourth, fifth, and sixth chakras. Sensory and motor nerves in the brachial plexus are stimulated by positioning the joints and contracting the muscles that create the asanas. The inversions also affect the autonomic nervous system, increasing parasympathetic output. This can temporarily decrease heart rate and blood pressure. Do these poses at the end of your session to prepare the body for Savasana (Corpse Pose).

The following asanas can be practiced from the standing version of Vinyasa Flow; they follow the same breathing sequence.

1. Take one full breath in Tadasana. Inhale and raise the arms to Urdhva Hastasana.

2. Exhale into Uttanasana. Extend the spine and look up on an inhale.

3. Exhale into Chaturanga.

4. Inhale into Upward Dog.

5. Exhale into Downward Dog.

6A. Exhale and jump or step forward to wrap the legs around the arms to move into Bhujapidasana (Shoulder-Pressing Pose). Press down with the hands and straighten the elbows. Squeeze the arms with the legs to create a bandha.

7. Then exhale and jump or step back into Chaturanga.

8. Inhale into Upward Dog.

9. Exhale into Downward Dog and rest there for five breaths.

10. Inhale and jump or step forward to Ardha Uttanasana (Half-Intense Forward-Bending Pose), lifting the chest and looking forward.

11. Then exhale into full Uttanasana. Hold this pose for a few breaths more after inversions. This allows the cardiovascular system to re-acclimate and helps to avoid light-headedness.

12. Inhale and extend the back to rise up into Urdhva Hastasana.

13. Exhale and lower the arms to Tadasana. Rest for a moment or two and then repeat the flow, integrating the next pose.

A

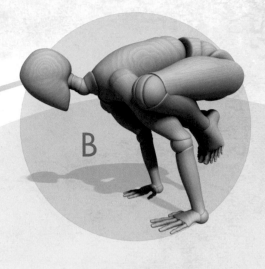

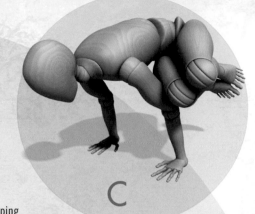

6B. Incorporate Bakasana into the sequence by jumping or stepping forward to place the upper shins on the outsides of the upper arms. Straighten the arms and squeeze against them by engaging the adductor muscles on the insides of the legs. This stabilizes the pose and creates a bandha.

6C. Then insert Parsva Bakasana, the turning version of Crow Pose. Press the side of the knee against the outer arm by engaging the abductor muscles on the side of the leg. This helps to turn the body into the twist.

6D. Go upside down into Handstand. You can leave the Vinyasa Flow for a moment and use a wall for support. Rest for a few breaths in Uttanasana after the pose and then repeat the flow.

6E. Go up into Pincha Mayurasana (Feathered Peacock Pose). Spread the weight over the entire forearm and lift the shoulders away from the ears. Then rest for a few breaths in Uttanasana. This allows the cardiovascular system to equilibrate. Repeat the Vinyasa.

6F. Finish this series with Headstand. With practice, you can learn to hold Sirsasana for longer than five breaths. Come down and rest in Child's Pose and then repeat the Vinyasa to balance the body. Do not practice Headstand if you have an injury or other pathology in the cervical spine region.

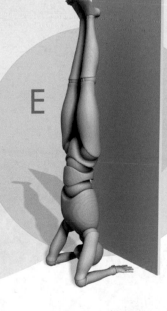

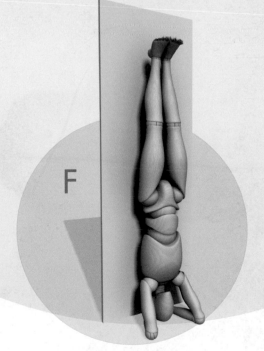

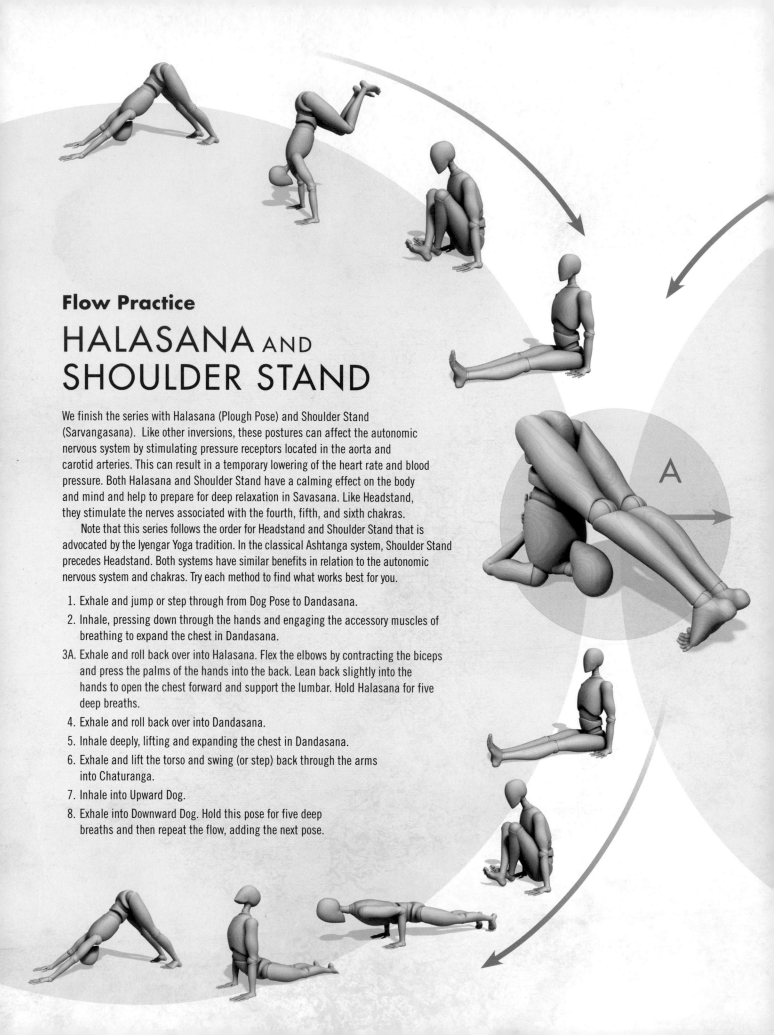

Flow Practice

HALASANA AND SHOULDER STAND

We finish the series with Halasana (Plough Pose) and Shoulder Stand (Sarvangasana). Like other inversions, these postures can affect the autonomic nervous system by stimulating pressure receptors located in the aorta and carotid arteries. This can result in a temporary lowering of the heart rate and blood pressure. Both Halasana and Shoulder Stand have a calming effect on the body and mind and help to prepare for deep relaxation in Savasana. Like Headstand, they stimulate the nerves associated with the fourth, fifth, and sixth chakras.

Note that this series follows the order for Headstand and Shoulder Stand that is advocated by the Iyengar Yoga tradition. In the classical Ashtanga system, Shoulder Stand precedes Headstand. Both systems have similar benefits in relation to the autonomic nervous system and chakras. Try each method to find what works best for you.

1. Exhale and jump or step through from Dog Pose to Dandasana.
2. Inhale, pressing down through the hands and engaging the accessory muscles of breathing to expand the chest in Dandasana.
3A. Exhale and roll back over into Halasana. Flex the elbows by contracting the biceps and press the palms of the hands into the back. Lean back slightly into the hands to open the chest forward and support the lumbar. Hold Halasana for five deep breaths.
4. Exhale and roll back over into Dandasana.
5. Inhale deeply, lifting and expanding the chest in Dandasana.
6. Exhale and lift the torso and swing (or step) back through the arms into Chaturanga.
7. Inhale into Upward Dog.
8. Exhale into Downward Dog. Hold this pose for five deep breaths and then repeat the flow, adding the next pose.

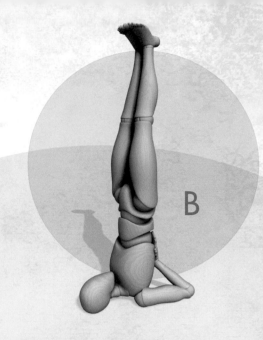

B

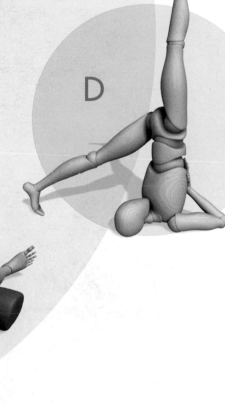

C

D

3B. Roll over into Halasana and then exhale and lift the legs into Shoulder Stand. Lean back into the hands and contract the biceps to bend the elbows; press the hands into the back and open the chest forward. Leaning back into the hands has the added benefit of taking the pressure off the cervical spine. Maintain the pose for five breaths in the beginning; build up to holding it longer with practice. Exhale down and back into Halasana; inhale and then exhale to roll out into Dandasana. Follow the flow as described on the previous page.

3C. Roll over into Halasana and then walk the feet around to the side, taking Parsva Halasana, the turning version of Plough Pose. Note that the feet will be uneven, with the outside foot further away from the body. Bend the knee to bring this foot in line with the inside foot; fix it on the mat and then straighten the knee. Note how this balances the pelvis. Repeat on the other side and then roll back into the Vinyasa Flow.

3D. Come up into Shoulder Stand from Halasana and then flex one hip to take Eka Pada Sarvangasana (One-Legged Shoulder Stand). Press the hands into the back and expand the chest. Then create a bandha by engaging the psoas on the side of the flexing hip and the gluteus maximus on the side with the leg in the air. This stabilizes the pose. Hold for five breaths and then return to Shoulder Stand. Repeat on the other side. Return to Halasana and then enter the flow.

3E. Lie down in Savasana. Place a folded blanket under the head to support it with the neck in a neutral or slightly flexed position. This is a gentle form of jalandhara bandha. You can also place a bolster under the knees, as shown. Let the arms and legs fall out to the side and turn the palms to face upward. This aids to passively open the chest. Close the eyes and sink into the floor. Completely relax and let go. Stay in Savasana for five to ten minutes—or more if you have time.

E

STANDING
POSES

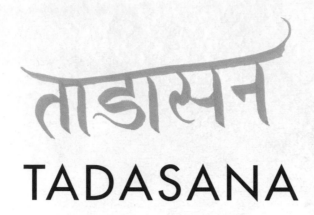

TADASANA

MOUNTAIN POSE

TADASANA IS THE KEYSTONE OF THE STANDING POSTURES. WE USE IT AS A physical barometer, a place of return between the standing poses where we can assess how the body feels after the preceding asana. Use the principle of co-activation in Tadasana. Spread the weight of the body evenly across the feet. Begin by pressing the back part of the heels into the floor. Then distribute the weight across the forefoot, from the balls of the feet toward the outer edges. Work your way up the legs, extending the knees by lifting the kneecaps. Align the bones of the legs, the femurs and tibias, and avoid hyperextending or "locking" the knees. This can cause misalignment of the leg bones. If you tend to hyperextend, contract the hamstrings to bend the knees and realign the femurs and tibias. Balance internal and external rotation of the femurs; similarly balance abduction (the force that draws the legs apart) with adduction (the force that draws the legs together) to create a sense of stability and stillness in the pose. Move the energy up to the pelvis, and stabilize the pelvis by co-activating the hip flexors and extensors. Balance extension and flexion of the lumbar spine, and gently engage the abdominal muscles to prevent the lower ribs from bulging forward. Align the vertebral column so that the spine assumes its natural curvature and "perches" effortlessly over the pelvis. For the Urdhva Hasta version of the pose, extend the elbows to lift the arms overhead. Draw the shoulders away from the ears and down the back to free the neck; allow the head to tilt back and the eyes to gaze upward.

BASIC JOINT POSITIONS

- The knees extend.
- The hips are neutral.
- The shoulders adduct in Tadasana.
- The shoulders flex in Urdhva Hastasana.
- The elbows extend.

- The cervical spine is neutral in Tadasana.
- The cervical spine extends in Urdhva Hastasana.
- The shoulder blades adduct and depress slightly.

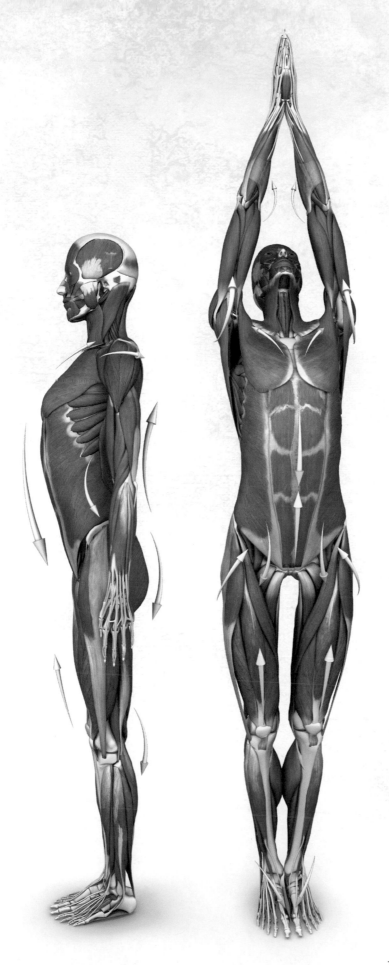

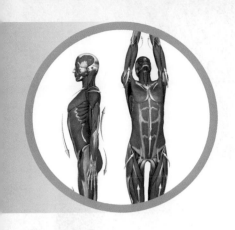

Tadasana Preparation

Internal forces, such as our mental state, influence our posture. For example, if we feel fatigued, defeated, or depressed, we might stand in Tadasana with slumped shoulders and a collapsed chest. Conversely, the form that we create with Tadasana influences our mental state. Bring the feet together and straighten the legs. Draw the shoulders back and down to open the chest. Straighten the arms. This relaxed yet open position counteracts a defeated and slumped posture in both body and mind.

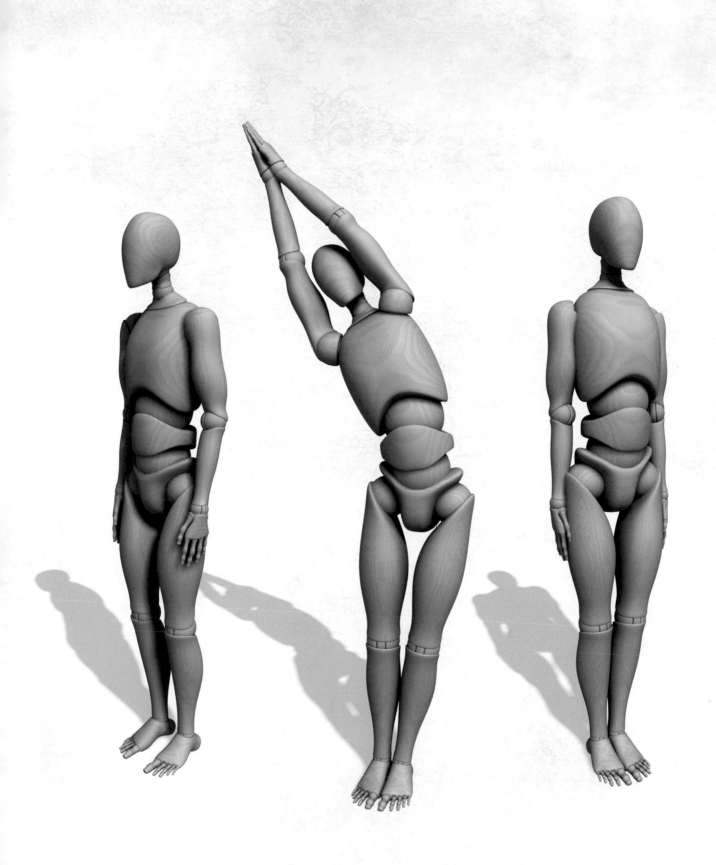

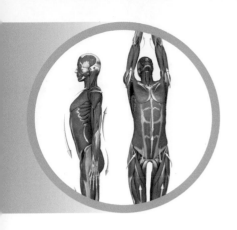

STEP 1 Lift the back and open the pelvic region using the posterior kinetic chain, a group of muscles, tendons, and ligaments on the back side of the body. Engage the erector spinae to extend the spine from the pelvis to the base of the skull, and activate the quadratus lumborum by gently arching the back to lift and support the lumbar region. Begin to balance the position of the pelvis by engaging the gluteus maximus; this muscle tilts the pelvis back and down into retroversion. It also extends and externally rotates the femurs. The gluteus minimus is a small muscle deep to the other buttocks muscles; visualize it contracting to stabilize the head of the femur bones in the hip sockets.

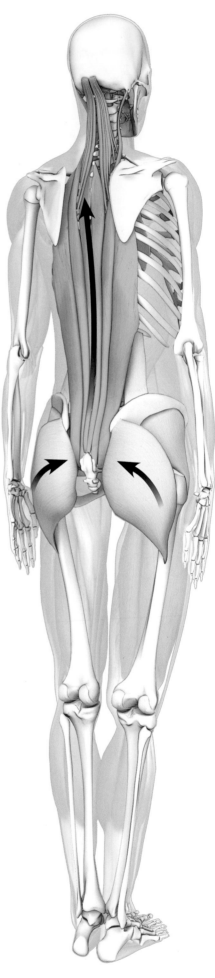

STEP 2 Engage the rectus abdominis to draw the ribcage downward, gently compressing the abdominal contents and stabilizing the lumbar spine. Activate the psoas major in combination with the iliacus and pectineus to tilt the pelvis slightly forward (anteversion) and balance the action of the gluteus maximus described in Step 1. The combined actions of the hip flexors and hip extensors bring the pelvis into a neutral position, neither tilted forward nor backward, but sitting like a bowl perched over the legs.

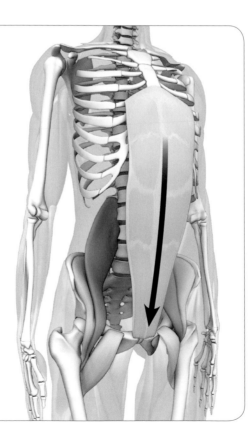

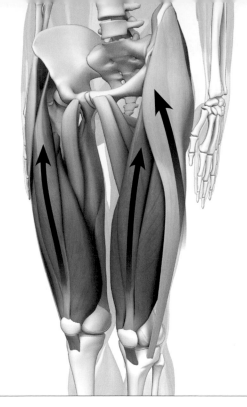

▶ STEP 3 Straighten the knees by engaging the quadriceps. One part of the quadriceps, the rectus femoris, crosses the hip joint and attaches to the pelvis, synergizing the psoas in tilting the pelvis forward. Contract the adductor muscles along the inner thighs to draw the femurs together. In Step 1 the gluteus maximus externally rotates the femurs. Use the gluteus medius and tensor fascia lata to balance this action by internally rotating the thighs. A cue for this is to attempt to drag the feet apart while engaging the adductor group.

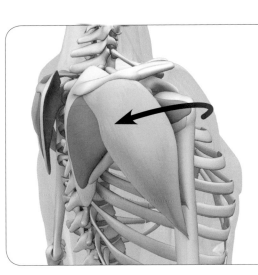

STEP 4 Activate the posterior deltoids and the infraspinatus and teres minor muscles of the rotator cuff to turn the shoulders outward at the glenohumeral joint and open the chest.

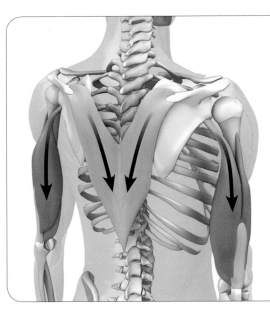

STEP 5 Engage the lower third of the trapezius to draw the shoulder blades down and away from the ears. Straighten the elbows by activating the triceps. Note how engaging the long head of the triceps (which originates from the shoulder blade) synergizes the action of the lower trapezius.

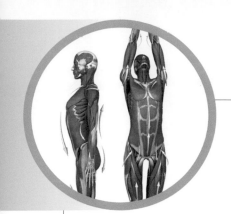

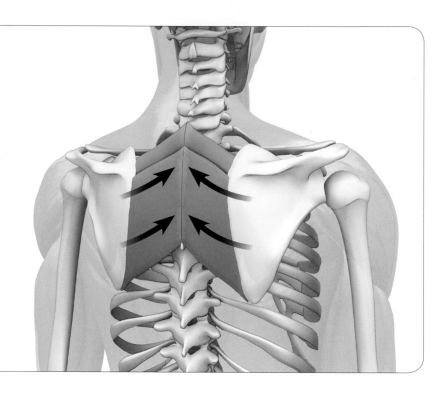

STEP 6 Draw the shoulder blades toward the midline and stabilize them in this position by engaging the rhomboids major and minor. This action opens the anterior (front) chest.

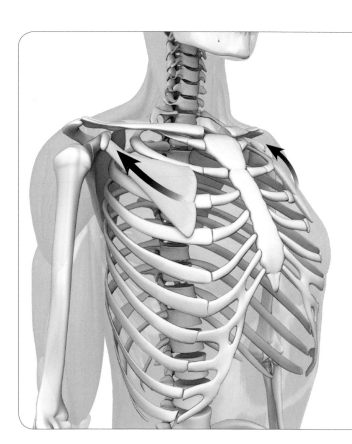

STEP 7 In Step 6 we engaged the rhomboids to stabilize the shoulder blades in place. Now activate the pectoralis minor to lift the lower ribcage and expand the chest. The cue for this is to draw the scapulae back, and then attempt to roll the shoulders forward. This is the basis for what is known as *bucket handle breathing* and is an example of using the accessory muscles of breathing to increase inspiratory volume. Rolling the shoulders forward mimics the usual action of the pectoralis minor and causes it to contract. Because the scapulae cannot move, the shoulders do not roll forward, and the force of this contraction is transmitted to the origin of the muscle on the ribcage, lifting it. This is an example of closed chain contraction of a muscle, whereby the origin rather than the insertion moves.

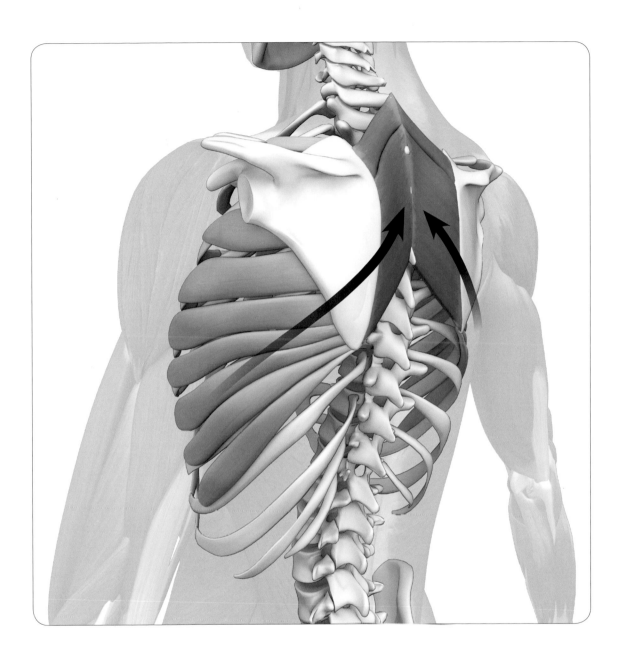

STEP 8 Normally we use the serratus anterior to draw the scapulae away from the midline, but here we use it to open the ribcage. With the scapulae stabilized in Step 6, visualize pressing your hands outward into a doorway to recruit the serratus anterior. The shoulder blades will not move, but the force of this contraction will be transmitted to the origin of the serratus anterior on the upper ribcage, lifting the chest. This is another example of using closed chain contraction to increase lung ventilation in a yoga pose.

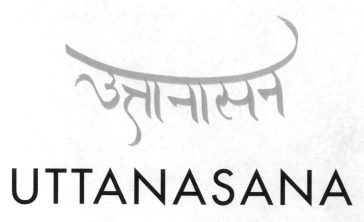

UTTANASANA

INTENSE FORWARD-BENDING POSE

UTTANASANA IS A STANDING POSE AND A FORWARD BEND THAT FUNCTIONS TO lengthen the hamstring and calf muscles, with a secondary stretch of the back. You can use a technique called triangulation to locate the focus of the stretch and deepen it. For example, activate the quadriceps to straighten the knees. This moves the hamstring insertions farther away from their origin on the ischial tuberosities (the sitting bones). Flex the trunk to draw the ischial tuberosities up and away from the hamstring insertions on the lower legs. To produce this action, simultaneously contract the hip and trunk flexors to draw the torso forward while engaging the quadriceps. These actions combine to move the origin and insertion of the hamstrings farther apart, "triangulating" the hamstrings and stretching the muscle. To add to this stretch, constrain your hands on the mat and attempt to drag them forward by bending the elbows; this draws the trunk further into flexion and exemplifies a secondary action contributing to the primary action of the pose. If you cannot reach the floor, grasp the backs of your knees or lower legs and bend the elbows. Because the hands are fixed in place, on the mat or holding the legs, the contractile force of the biceps draws the trunk deeper into flexion. This force is transmitted through the posterior kinetic chain to the pelvis, tilting it forward and lifting the ischial tuberosities, thereby augmenting the stretch of the hamstrings.

Remember that contracting the quadriceps creates reciprocal inhibition of the hamstrings, their antagonist, signaling the hamstrings to relax and move more deeply into the stretch. Experience this in Uttanasana by firmly engaging the quadriceps, and note how the sensation of the stretch changes.

BASIC JOINT POSITIONS

- The hips flex.
- The trunk flexes.
- The femurs internally rotate (slightly).
- The knees extend.

- The cervical spine is neutral.
- The shoulders flex overhead.
- The elbows flex.
- The forearms pronate.

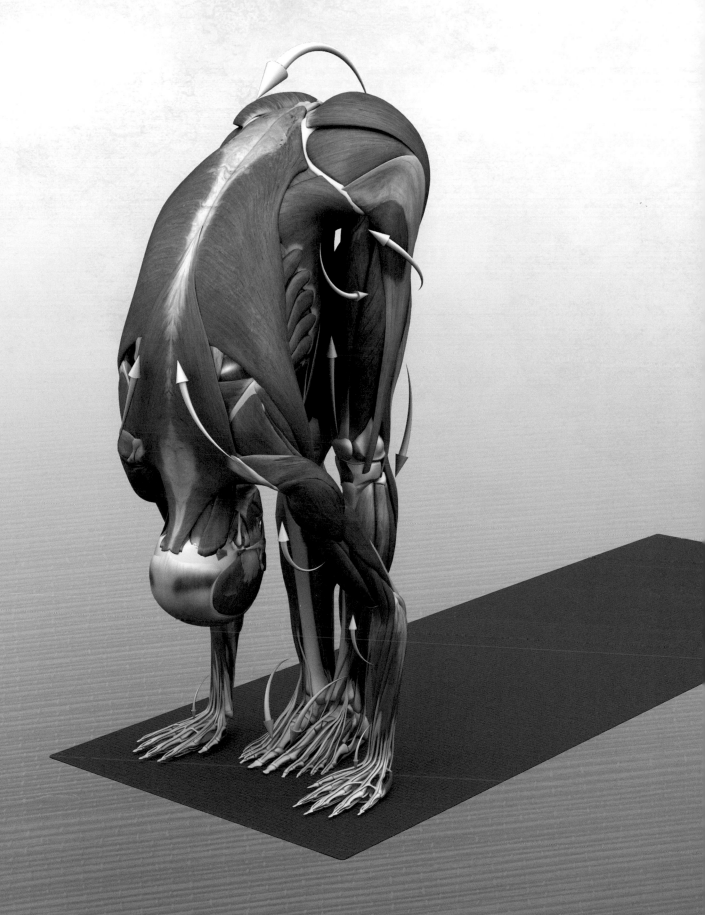

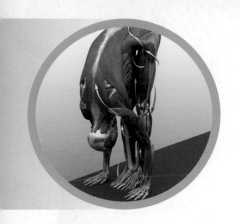

Uttanasana Preparation

Tightness in the hamstrings and/or back muscles can limit the depth of the forward bend in Uttanasana. At first, allow the muscles to acclimate to being stretched by resting on a chair with the knees bent. This releases the hamstrings at their origin on the ischial tuberosities.

Then gradually straighten the knees by activating the quadriceps. As your flexibility increases, you can draw the trunk toward the thighs with the knees slightly bent. Holding the trunk in this position, engage the quadriceps to straighten the knees, and feel the stretch in the hamstrings. If the back is more flexible but the hamstrings are tight, then fold forward (flexion) with the knees slightly bent. You can also prepare the body for Uttanasana by using a forward bend such as Paschimottanasana (Intense Stretch to the West Pose) to lengthen the posterior kinetic chain.

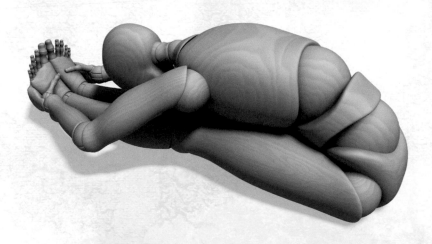

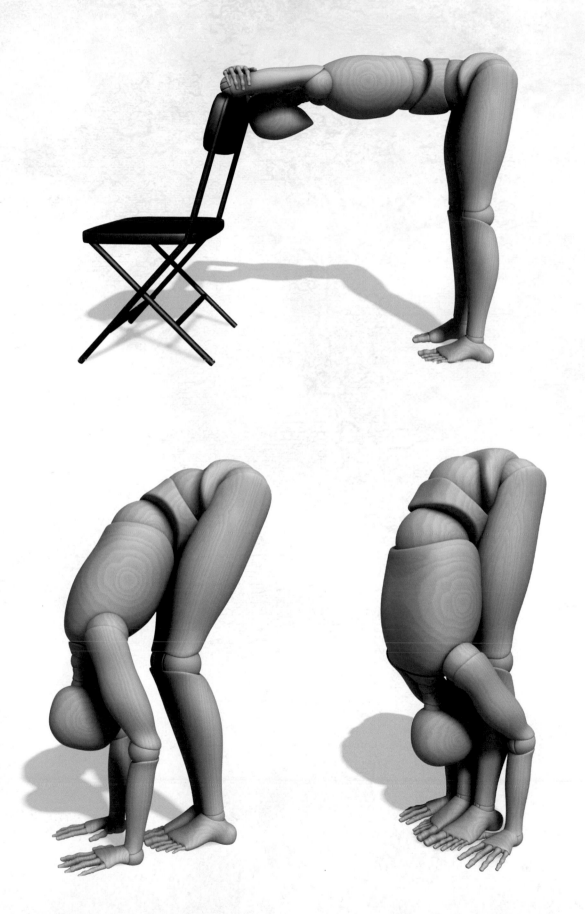

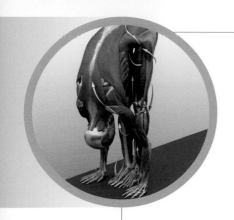

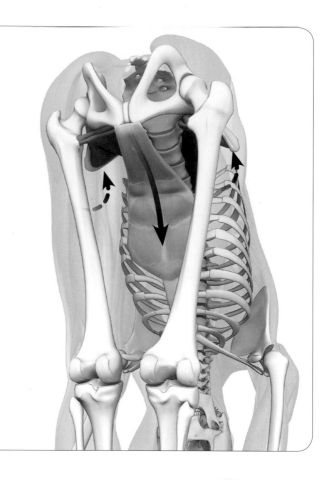

STEP 1 Flex the trunk by activating the rectus abdominis. This creates reciprocal inhibition of the lower back muscles, signaling them to relax. Tilt the pelvis forward by contracting the hip flexors, including the psoas, pectineus, and anterior adductor muscles. This signals the hip extensors (the gluteals) to relax.

▶ **STEP 2** Activate the quadriceps to straighten the knees. The tensor fascia lata synergizes this action when the knees are straight. Bear in mind that when we stretch a muscle, we also pull on its attachments and passively produce the same movements as when we contract the muscle. Pulling on the gluteus maximus thus externally rotates the thigh. Engaging the tensor fascia lata also turns the femurs in slightly. The cue for this action is to attempt to gently drag the feet apart. Use this action to adjust the femurs, so that the kneecaps point forward symmetrically. The feet do not move, but the femurs turn inward with this cue. The gluteus minimus is also pictured here. This muscle synergizes hip flexion when the femur is flexed. Use the image to help visualize the muscle engaging.

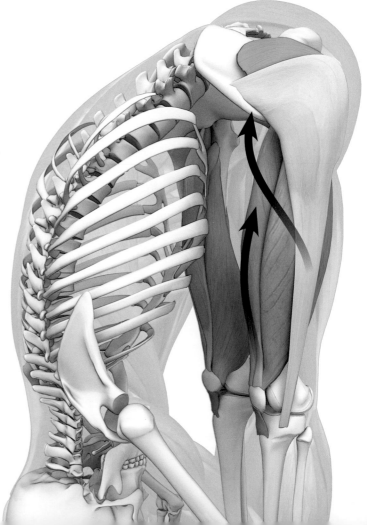

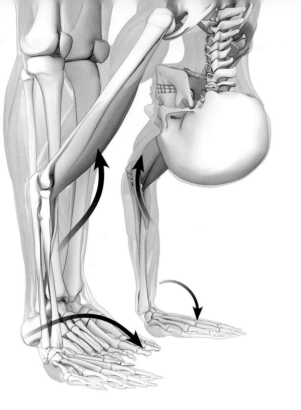

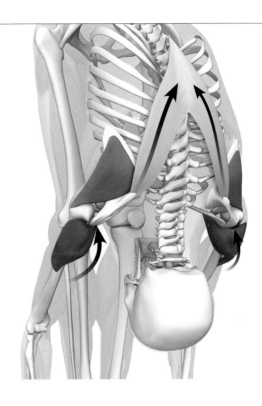

◄STEP 3 Pronate the forearms to press the mounds of the palms of the hands (the fleshy area at the base of the fingers) into the mat. With the hands fixed on the floor, attempt to bend the elbows by contracting the biceps. This draws the trunk toward the thighs.

STEP 4 Draw the shoulders away from the ears by activating the lower third of the trapezius. Keep the hands fixed on the floor, as described in Step 3, and attempt to drag the hands forward by contracting the anterior deltoids. This synergizes the action of the biceps in the previous step to flex the trunk more deeply. Remember to activate the quadriceps when applying these secondary actions so that you create reciprocal inhibition of the hamstrings, helping them to relax into the stretch.

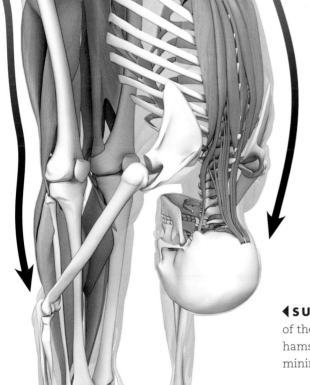

◄SUMMARY The steps described above stretch the muscles of the posterior kinetic chain, including the gastrocnemius, hamstrings, gluteus maximus, and posterior portions of the gluteus minimus, quadratus lumborum, and erector spinae.

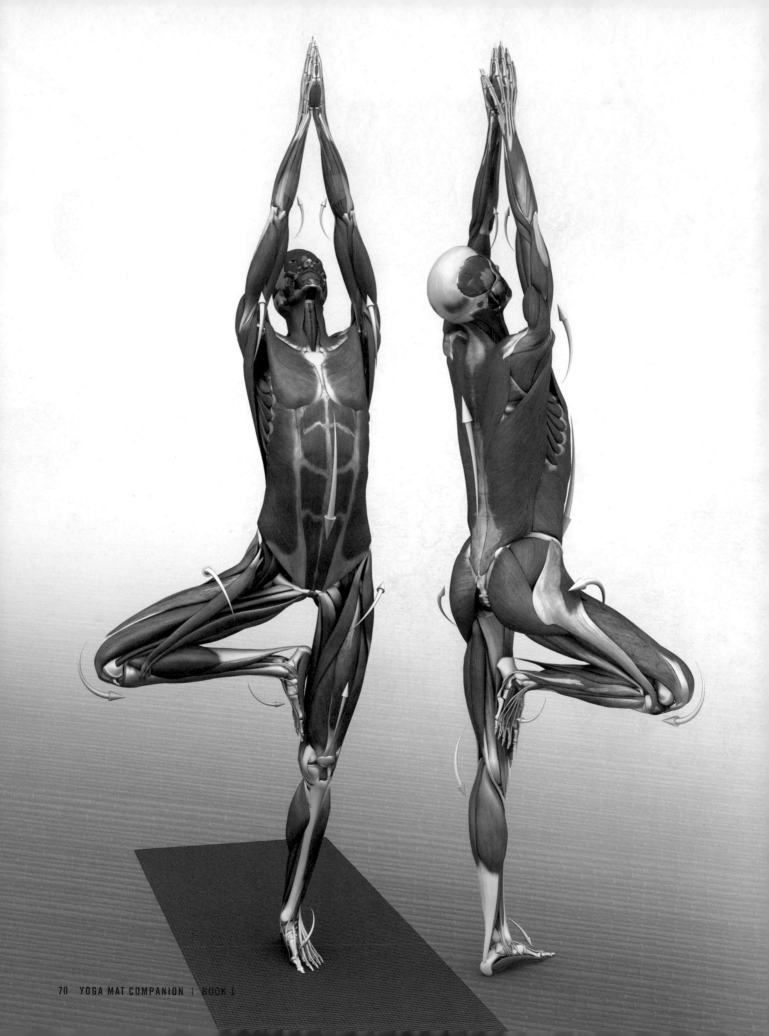

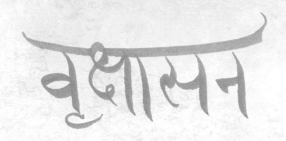

VRKSASANA

TREE POSE

SEVERAL STORIES TAKE PLACE SIMULTANEOUSLY IN THIS POSE. VRKSASANA IS both a balancing pose and, secondarily, a hip opener. It also contains elements of movement that ascend while others remain rooted into the ground. Apply the concepts used in Tadasana to the standing leg in Tree Pose, beginning with the foot. Remember that changes in the pressure of the standing foot are transmitted to the pelvic core and vice versa. Connect the two regions in the mind. Try the pose in a setting where you can place the hand on a wall for balance (even if you can balance without the wall). Then press the ball of the foot into the mat, and spread the weight evenly across the sole of the foot. Straighten the knee by activating the quadriceps, and be alert for hyperextension. Bend the knee to lower the center of gravity (creating stability), and then straighten back up.

Look at the subplot of the bent leg: the hamstrings activate to bend the knee; the adductor group presses the sole of the foot into the inner thigh of the standing leg; and the hip abductors, gluteals, and deep external rotators contract to draw the knee back and externally rotate the femur. The balance of the pelvis results from the interplay of various muscles that move the hip—the adductors, abductors, extensors, flexors, and rotators. Move up the body to the back and balance the activation of the erector spinae and quadratus lumborum with that of the abdominal muscles on the front body. Draw the shoulder blades toward the midline and down the back. Then activate the pectoralis minor and serratus anterior muscles to lift the chest. Let the head drop back in a relaxed fashion.

BASIC JOINT POSITIONS

- The standing hip is neutral.
- The standing knee extends.
- The raised-leg hip flexes, abducts, and externally rotates.
- The raised-leg knee flexes.
- The back extends slightly.
- The shoulders abduct and flex overhead.
- The elbows extend.
- The palms flex slightly.

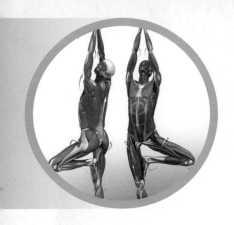

Vrksasana Preparation

Use a chair or wall for balance. Place the hands on the hips and then in prayer position on the chest. Finally, raise the arms overhead. If you lose your balance, bend your standing leg to lower the center of gravity. Practice poses like Baddha Konasana (Bound Angle Pose) to prepare the hip of the lifted leg for flexion, abduction, and external rotation.

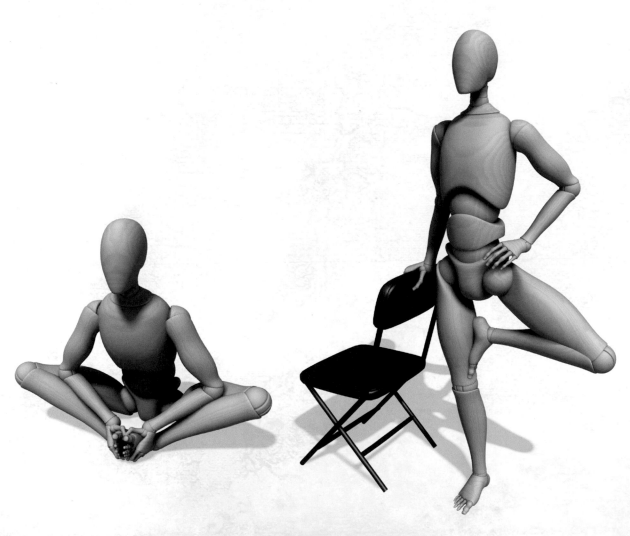

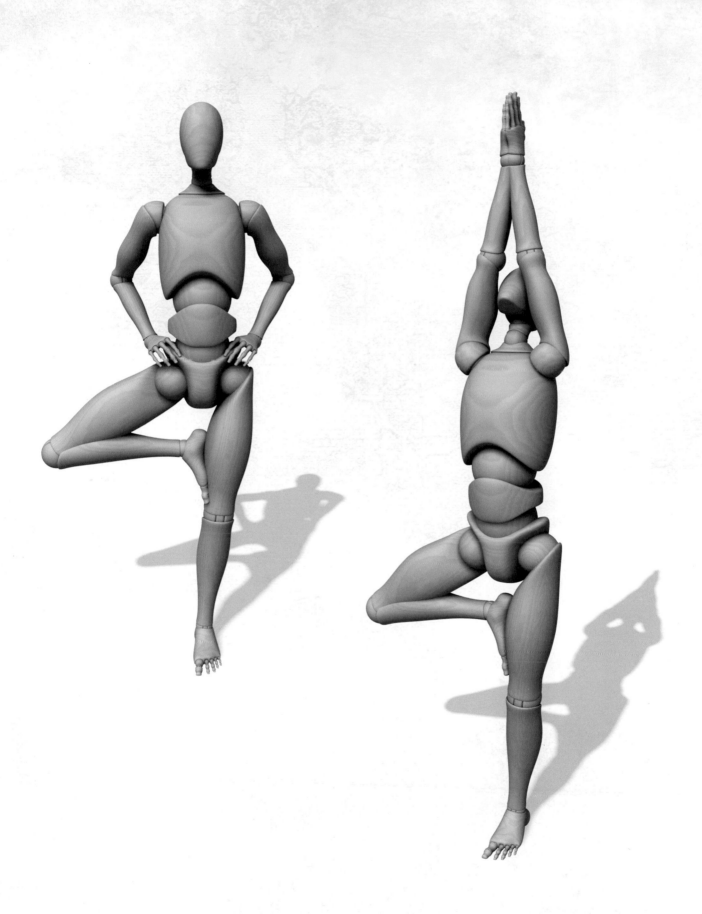

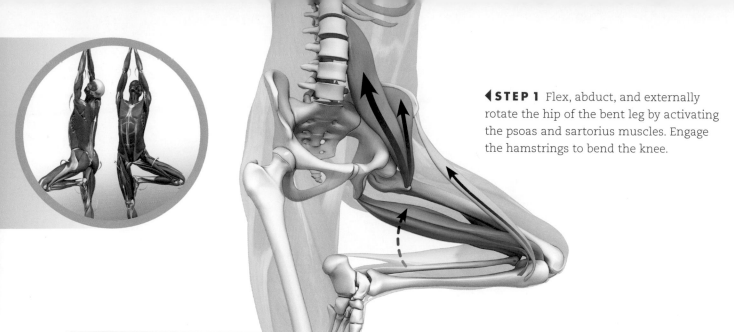

◀ **STEP 1** Flex, abduct, and externally rotate the hip of the bent leg by activating the psoas and sartorius muscles. Engage the hamstrings to bend the knee.

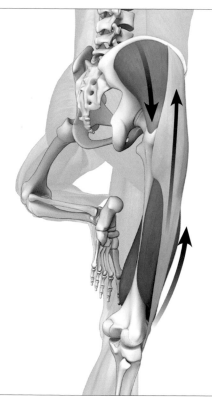

STEP 2 Activate the quadriceps to straighten the standing leg. The gluteus medius automatically contracts when you balance on one leg. You can see from the inset that if the gluteus medius did not activate, the body would shift over and beyond the standing leg and the pelvis would tilt excessively. The bent-leg foot pressing into the thigh stabilizes the standing leg. The tensor fascia lata is a synergist of the gluteus medius in this pose. Visualize this muscle contracting to refine balance and stability. Additionally, the tensor fascia lata works to extend the knee, so it is also a synergist of the quadriceps.

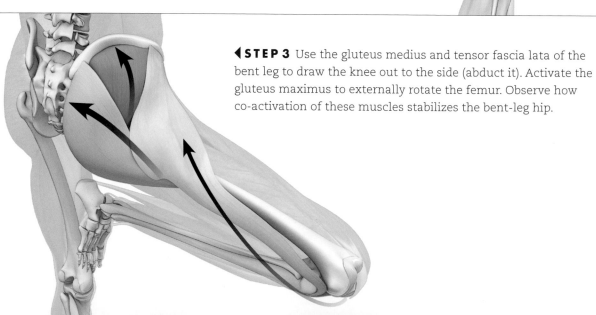

◀ **STEP 3** Use the gluteus medius and tensor fascia lata of the bent leg to draw the knee out to the side (abduct it). Activate the gluteus maximus to externally rotate the femur. Observe how co-activation of these muscles stabilizes the bent-leg hip.

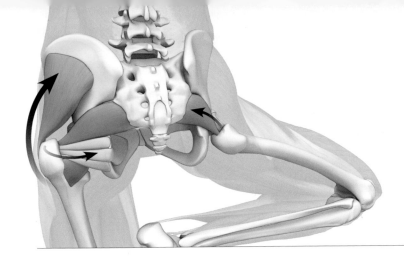

▲ **STEP 4** Contract the deep external rotators to open the hips and create space in the front of the pelvis. Notice the gluteus minimus in this pose. This muscle is deep to the gluteus medius and has different functions, depending on whether the hip is flexed, extended, or neutral. In Vrksasana, the standing hip is neutral, so the gluteus minimus works to stabilize the ball of the hip joint in the socket. Also look at the interplay between the gluteus minimus and the deep external rotators illustrated here. This combination of muscles stabilizes the hip of the standing leg.

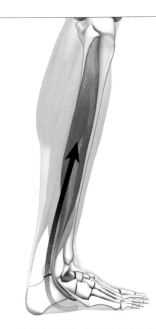

STEP 5 Activate the peroneus longus and brevis muscles on the side of the standing leg to spread the weight across the ball of the foot. Balancing on the standing-leg foot shows a complex interplay among the muscles that evert the foot and press the ball of the foot down, those that invert the foot, and those that flex and extend the ankle. The tibialis posterior balances the eversion force from the peronei and dynamizes the longitudinal foot arch. The muscles of the toes also contribute to stability in the pose.

▶ **SUMMARY** Connect the various parts of the body, from the foundation formed by the standing foot through to the palms of the hands. Engage the muscles of the ankle and foot to stabilize the foot, the quadriceps to extend the knee, and the abductors (the gluteus medius and tensor fascia lata) to stabilize the pelvis. The pelvis connects to the spine through the erector spinae. Engage the deltoids to lift the arms and the infraspinati to externally rotate the upper arm bones. Draw the shoulders away from the ears with the lower third of the trapezius. Contract the forearm pronators to counter this outward rotation and create a helical force through the elbows. Press the palms of the hands together evenly.

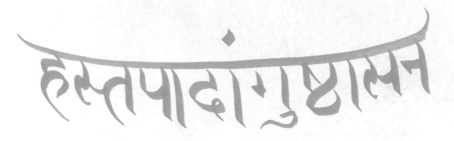

UTTHITA HASTA PADANGUSTHASANA

STANDING BIG-TOE HOLD POSE

UTTHITA HASTA PADANGUSTHASANA USES MANY OF THE SAME PRINCIPLES THAT apply to Tree Pose. Again we have several plots involved in the story of this pose—balancing on one leg, intensely stretching the lifted leg, extending the back to maintain the body erect, and contracting the muscles of the arm to lift the foot. Even the action of the big toe that is being held is a subplot. Then there is the mental aspect of staying calm to maintain balance. This is aided by focusing on the breath—the underlying story in all of the asanas. Balance the action of the peronei, which press the ball of the foot into the floor, with the action of the tibialis posterior, which spreads the weight across the sole of the foot. Essentially all of the lower leg and foot muscles help to create a firm foundation for the pose. The key to success in this posture is actively flexing the hip of the lifted leg. The tendency is to use the hand and arm to lift the foot. Instead, use the hip flexors to lift the leg and the arm as an adjunct to refine the lift.

BASIC JOINT POSITIONS

- The standing knee extends.
- The standing hip is in neutral.
- The raised knee extends.
- The raised hip flexes.

- The shoulder of the raised arm flexes.
- The back extends slightly to counterbalance reaching forward for the foot.

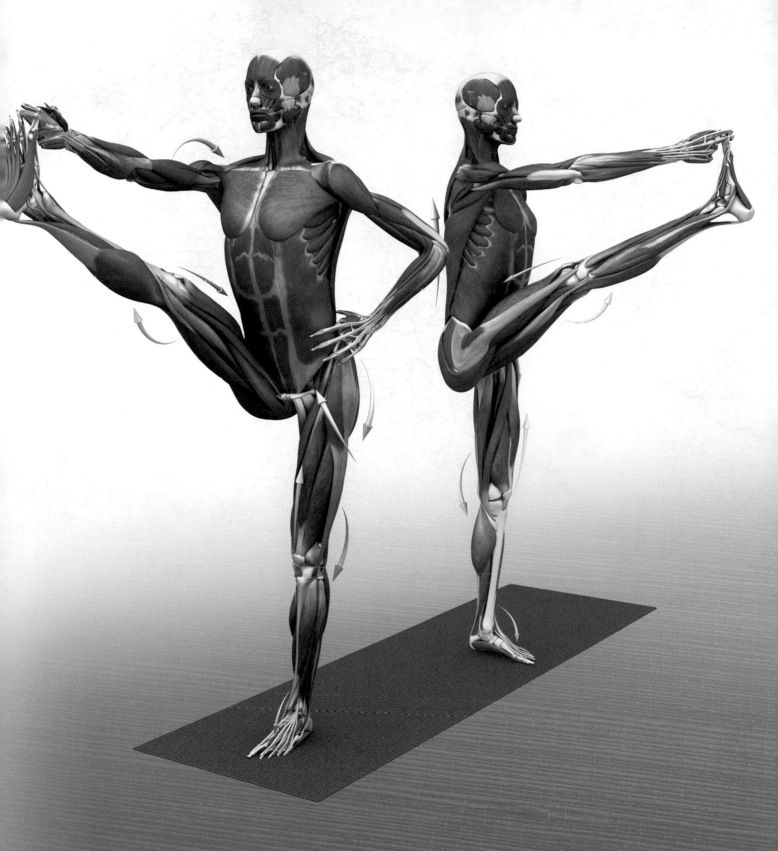

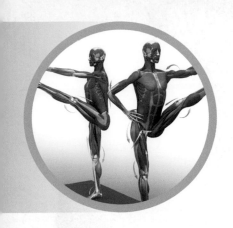

Utthita Hasta Padangusthasana Preparation

Use a wall to balance at first, and train yourself to lift the leg in the air by activating the hip flexors. In the beginning, bend the knee. Hold the knee in the air without using your hand. This trains the hip flexors to engage. Then wrap a belt around the foot to allow the leg to straighten. As you develop flexibility and balance, move away from the wall. Create stability by bending the standing leg to lower the center of gravity, and then work toward straightening the leg. You can also bend the leg in the air to release the hamstrings, and then work toward extending the knee of this leg. If you start to lose balance, bend both knees to regain stability.

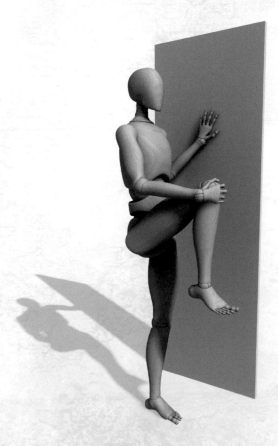

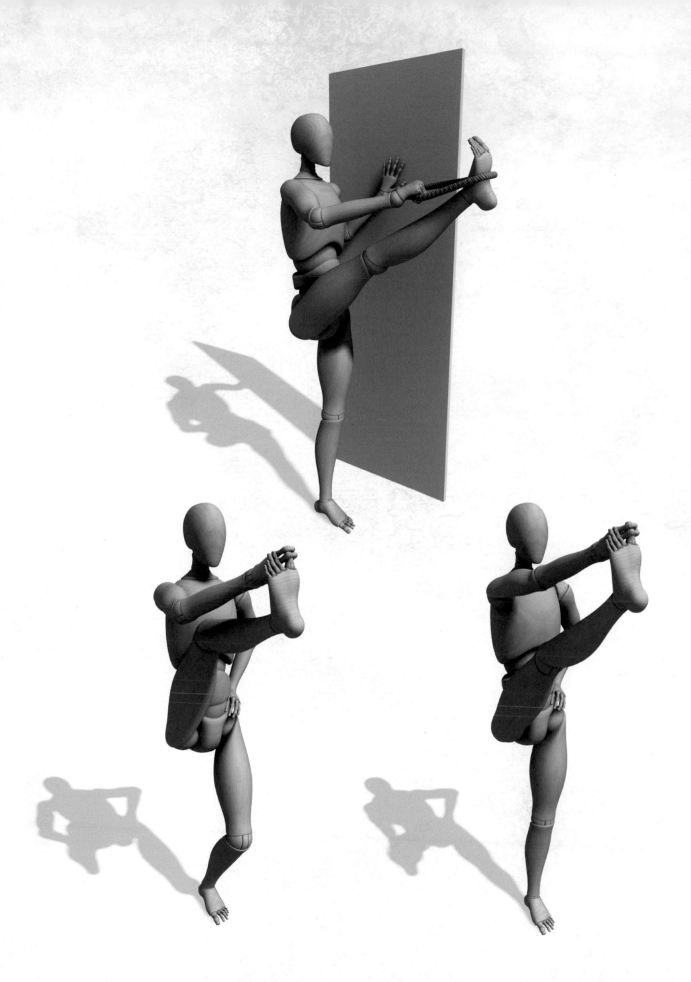

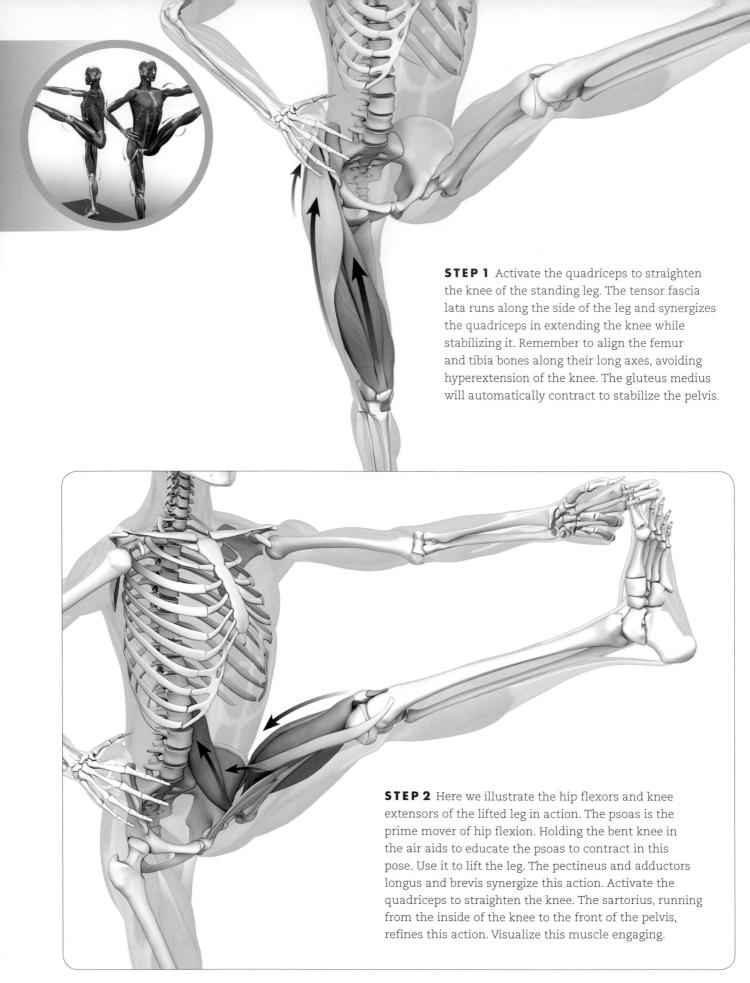

STEP 1 Activate the quadriceps to straighten the knee of the standing leg. The tensor fascia lata runs along the side of the leg and synergizes the quadriceps in extending the knee while stabilizing it. Remember to align the femur and tibia bones along their long axes, avoiding hyperextension of the knee. The gluteus medius will automatically contract to stabilize the pelvis.

STEP 2 Here we illustrate the hip flexors and knee extensors of the lifted leg in action. The psoas is the prime mover of hip flexion. Holding the bent knee in the air aids to educate the psoas to contract in this pose. Use it to lift the leg. The pectineus and adductors longus and brevis synergize this action. Activate the quadriceps to straighten the knee. The sartorius, running from the inside of the knee to the front of the pelvis, refines this action. Visualize this muscle engaging.

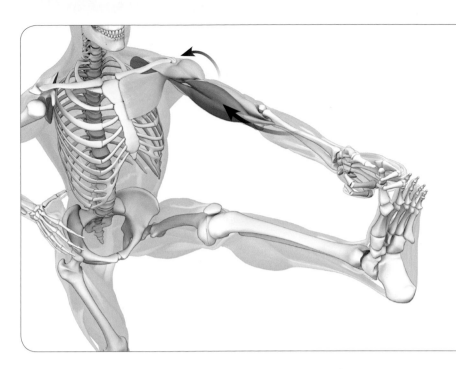

STEP 3 Now use the arm to lift the leg higher. Contract the upper sternoclavicular region of the pectoralis major and the anterior deltoid to lift the arm. To get a feel for engaging these muscles, press the palm of the hand against a wall and attempt to scrub it up toward the ceiling. Then return to the pose. Bend the elbow by activating the biceps and brachialis muscles. These actions raise the leg and augment the stretch of the gluteus maximus, hamstrings, and gastrocnemius.

STEP 4 There is a tendency to lean forward in this pose due to the pull of the raised-leg hamstrings and gluteus maximus on the structures of the posterior chain. Correct this by arching the lumbar to activate the erector spinae and by engaging the standing-leg buttocks, quadratus lumborum, and gluteus maximus. Note how this draws the foot that is held in the air higher and accentuates the stretch at the back of the leg.

SUMMARY In Utthita Hasta Padangusthasana, the main plot played out in the pose is the hamstring stretch of the lifted leg. The subplot, or secondary stretch, takes place at the gastrocnemius and gluteus maximus muscles.

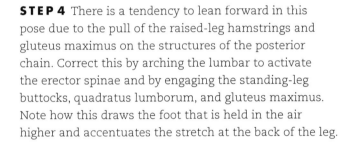
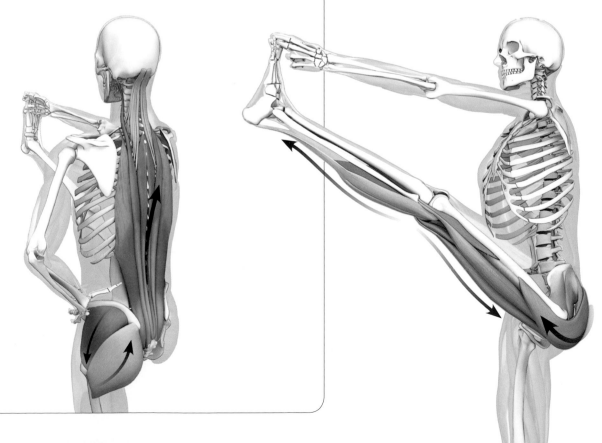

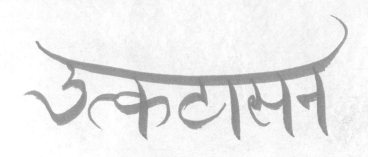

UTKATASANA

CHAIR POSE

UTKATASANA, LIKE VRKSASANA, USES THE CONCEPT OF SIMULTANEOUS ASCENT and descent. Several actions within the pose create this effect. Flex the hips to tilt the pelvis forward. Counteract this by engaging the buttocks muscles to tilt the pelvis downward from the back (into retroversion). Press the feet down evenly, beginning at the heels and then spreading the weight across the soles of the feet; squeeze the knees together. You will find this brings stability and balance to the pose. The combination of these actions creates the downward force of the lower body that is felt in Utkatasana. Ascend the upper body by activating the erector spinae and quadratus lumborum to lift the torso. Draw the shoulder blades toward the midline and down the back to open the chest upward. Raise the arms and straighten the elbows. Polish the pose by gently engaging the rectus abdominis to counteract any bulging forward of the ribcage.

BASIC JOINT POSITIONS

- The knees flex.
- The hips adduct and flex.
- The back extends.
- The shoulders flex overhead and externally rotate.

- The elbows extend.
- The forearms pronate.
- The cervical spine extends to tilt the head back.

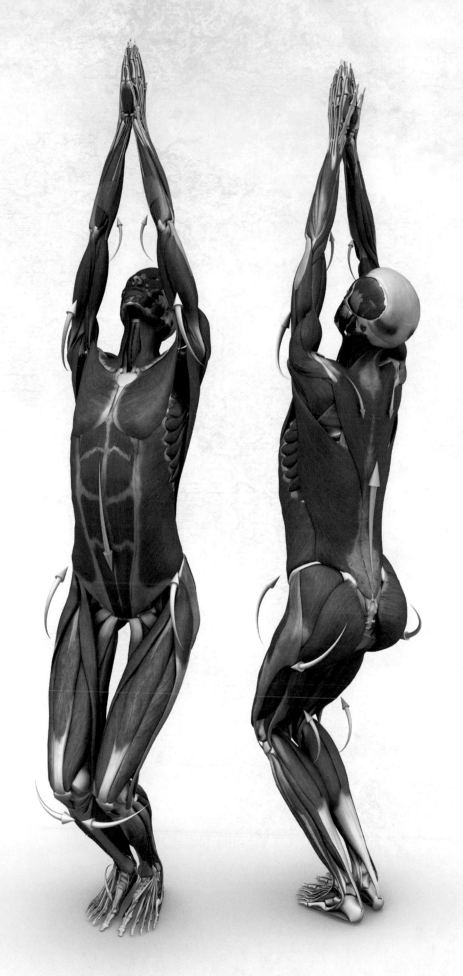

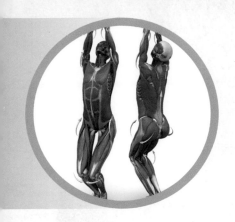

Utkatasana Preparation

Begin with the hands on the hips to lower the center of gravity. Draw the shoulder blades toward the midline of the back to open the chest. Bend the knees, and activate the adductor muscles to squeeze the inner knees together. Balance the forward and backward tilt of the pelvis and spread the weight of the body across the soles of the feet. Begin with more weight in your heels, so that gravity is directed through the center of the ankles rather than forward on the feet. Then raise the arms overhead, draw the shoulders down the back to free the neck, and tilt the head back to look up at the hands. You can use a chair to stretch the shoulder extensors. Place the elbows on the chair as shown, flex the trunk, and holding this position, press the elbows into the chair to create a facilitated stretch. Relax and flex the trunk deeper to open the shoulders. Then take Utkatasana and note how you can raise the arms further overhead.

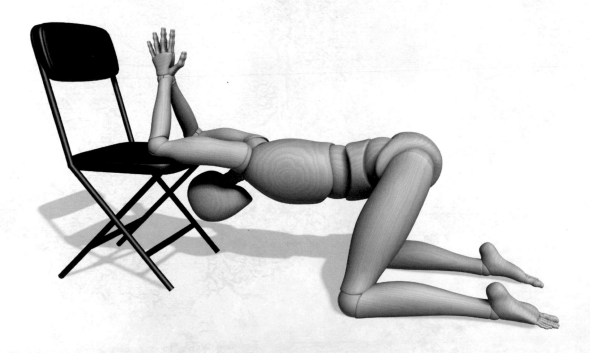

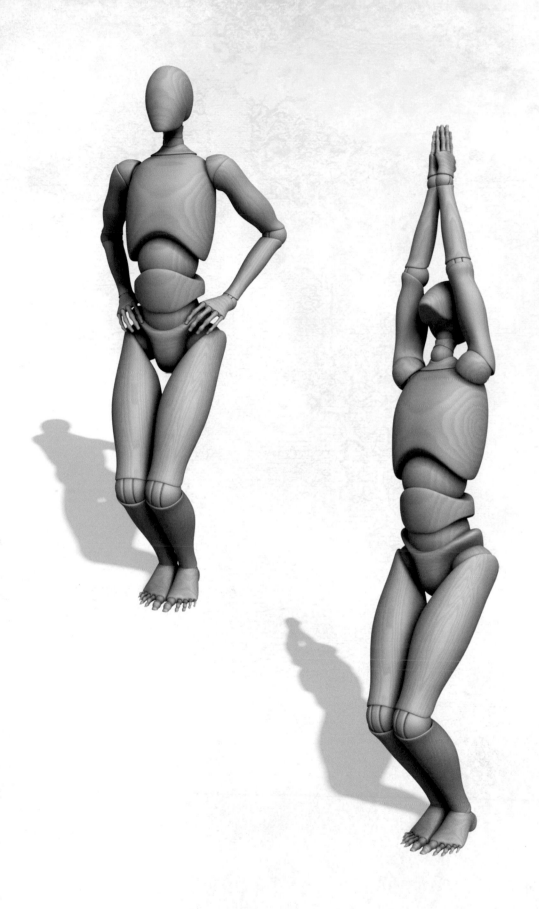

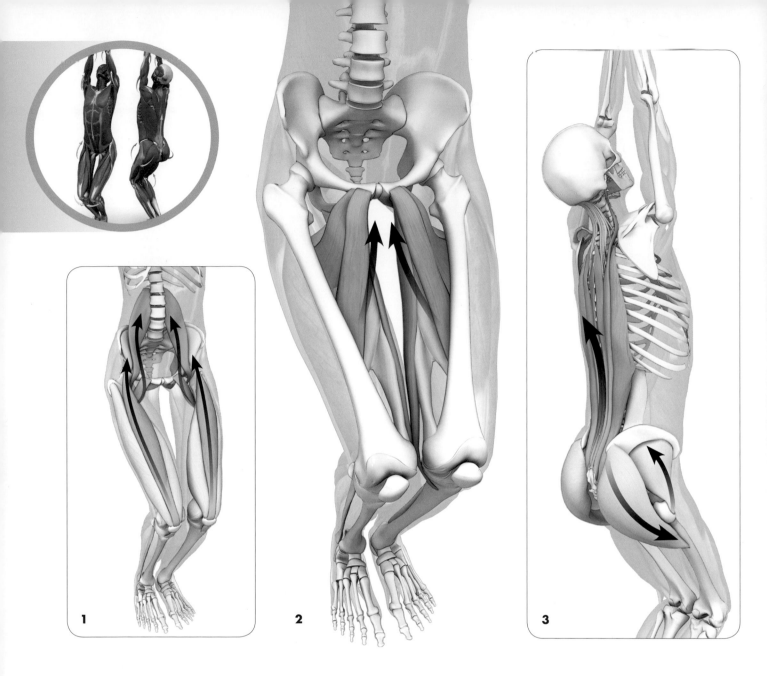

STEP 1 Activate the psoas and pectineus muscles to flex the hips. Bend the knees and stabilize the lower body by engaging the quadriceps. Note how one of the heads of the quadriceps, the rectus femoris, synergizes the hip flexors. This is because the muscle is polyarticular (it crosses more than one joint) and originates from the front of the pelvic bone. Visualize the rectus femoris in action in order to engage it.

STEP 2 Squeeze the knees together by activating the adductor group of muscles on the inner thighs. The more anteriorly placed muscles, the adductors longus and brevis, also help to tilt the pelvis forward.

STEP 3 Activate the gluteus maximus to tilt the pelvis downward and back, counterbalancing the forward tilt of the pelvis created by the hip flexors. Notice the gluteus minimus. This muscle synergizes flexion of the hips in this position. Lift the torso by contracting the erector spinae and quadratus lumborum.

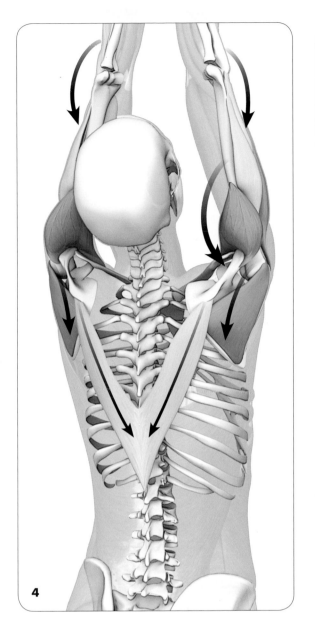

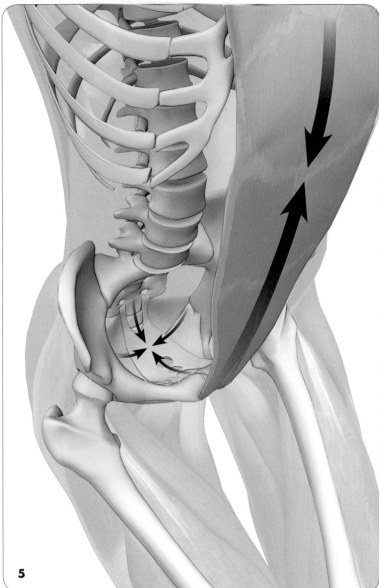

STEP 4 Lift the arms by activating the anterior (front) portion of the deltoids. Straighten the elbows by contracting the triceps, and externally rotate the shoulders by activating the infraspinatus. Engage the pectoralis minor and serratus anterior muscles (as in Tadasana) to expand the chest upward. Tilt the head back.

STEP 5 Complete the pose by contracting the rectus abdominis. This draws the ribcage down, stretching the intercostal muscles. It also increases intra-abdominal pressure and creates an "air bag" effect to stabilize the spine. Activate the muscles of the pelvic floor to create mula bandha. You can augment the force of contraction of the bandha by squeezing the knees together while engaging the muscles of the pelvic diaphragm. This action is referred to as recruitment.

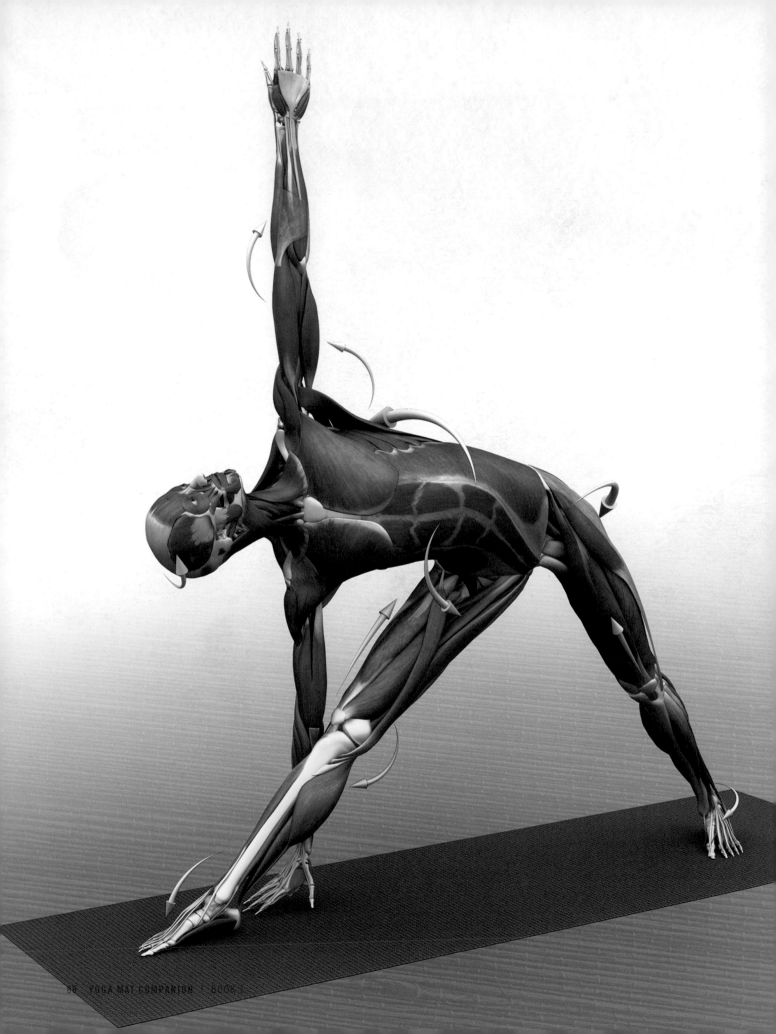

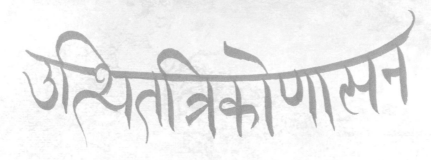

UTTHITA TRIKONASANA

EXTENDED TRIANGLE POSE

THE PRIMARY FOCUS OF TRIANGLE POSE IS THE STRETCH OF THE FRONT-LEG hamstrings. Contributing subplots, or secondary regions that stretch, include the upper side of the trunk and the back-leg hamstring and gastrocnemius muscles. The front of the pelvis also opens as the back hip externally rotates. Be aware of the feet in Trikonasana, spreading the body weight evenly across the soles. Activate the gluteal muscles and the quadriceps of the back leg by attempting to scrub the back foot away from the front. Because the foot remains fixed on the mat and cannot move, the force of this action is transmitted to the back of the knee on the rear leg, opening this region. Notice how straightening the curve of the upper-side back increases the stretch of the front-leg hamstrings. This is because engaging the upper-side quadratus lumborum muscle tilts the pelvis slightly forward, lifting the ischial tuberosities. Look at the arrow showing the rotation of the trunk upward, and see the connection of this movement to the hamstring muscles. The tendency is for the front knee to turn in as the body turns up. Counter this tendency by externally rotating the hip to keep the knee facing forward. Press the ball of the foot into the floor to create a helical force up the leg. This illustrates the principle of co-activating muscles to create stability.

BASIC JOINT POSITIONS

- The front knee extends.
- The back knee extends.
- The back foot rotates inward 30 degrees and supinates.
- The front foot rotates out 90 degrees.
- The trunk laterally flexes.

- The front hip flexes.
- The back hip extends and externally rotates.
- Both shoulders abduct.
- Both elbows extend fully.
- The cervical spine rotates the head to face upward.

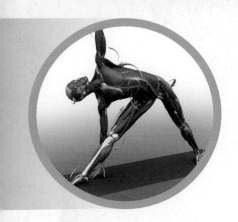

Utthita Trikonasana Preparation

Begin by turning the back foot in thirty degrees and the front foot out ninety degrees, so that a line drawn from the heel of the front foot transects the arch of the back foot. Activate the quadriceps to straighten the knees; contract the buttocks to open the front of the pelvis.

Next, bend the front knee and press the elbow onto the thigh by attempting to flex the trunk. This isolates and awakens the psoas muscle. You can also attempt to lift the leg up against the elbow (that is, attempt to flex the hip). Remember that the psoas flexes the trunk over the leg or flexes the leg toward the trunk. Recreating these movements against the resistance of the elbow awakens this muscle. When you activate the psoas, the pelvis tilts forward and the ischial tuberosities (the sitting bones) move backward. Feel how moving the origin of the hamstrings in this way increases the stretch. Straighten the front knee to stretch the hamstrings in the region of their insertions, and lower the trunk to deepen the pose.

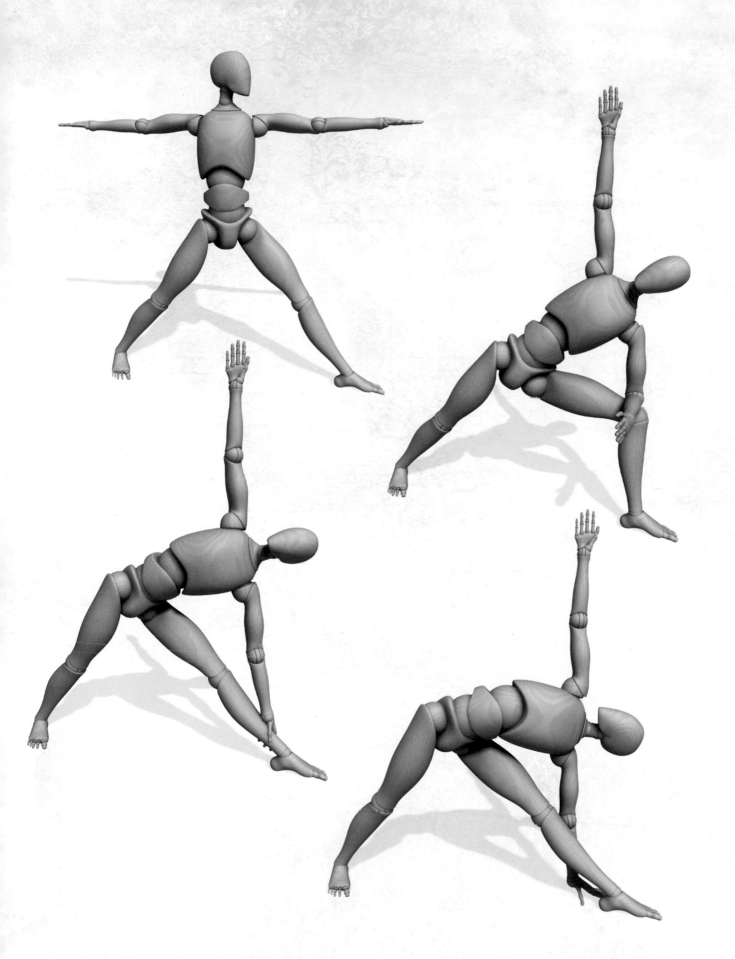

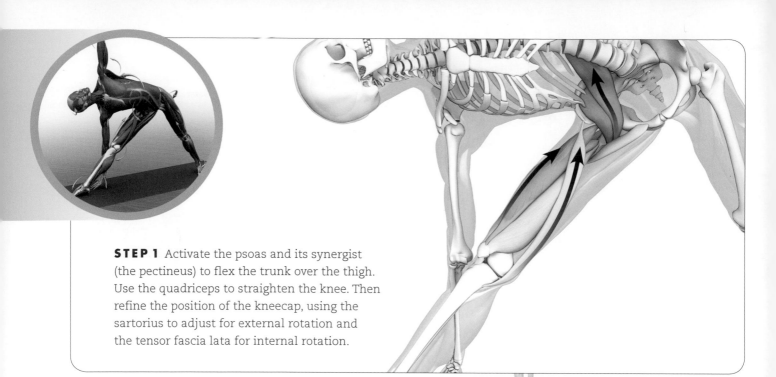

STEP 1 Activate the psoas and its synergist (the pectineus) to flex the trunk over the thigh. Use the quadriceps to straighten the knee. Then refine the position of the kneecap, using the sartorius to adjust for external rotation and the tensor fascia lata for internal rotation.

STEP 2 Turn the back foot inward and dorsiflex it by contracting the tibialis anterior. Activate the quadriceps to straighten the knee and the tensor fascia lata to internally rotate the thigh. This counterbalances external rotation of the thigh—an action of the back-leg gluteus maximus. Engage the gluteus medius by fixing the back foot on the mat, and attempt to drag it away from the front foot. The force of this action opens the back of the knee, creating a unique stretch of the hamstrings and other structures in this region.

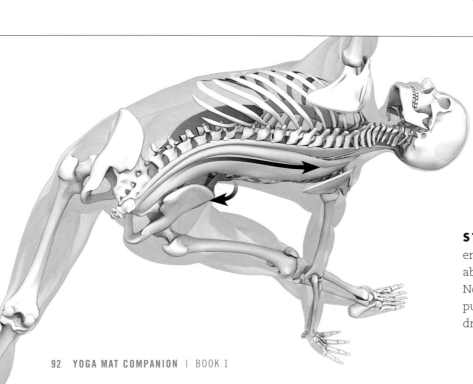

STEP 3 Engage the lower-side erector spinae muscles and oblique abdominals to laterally flex the trunk. Notice the effect of the erector spinae pulling on the pelvis and how this draws the sitting bones upward.

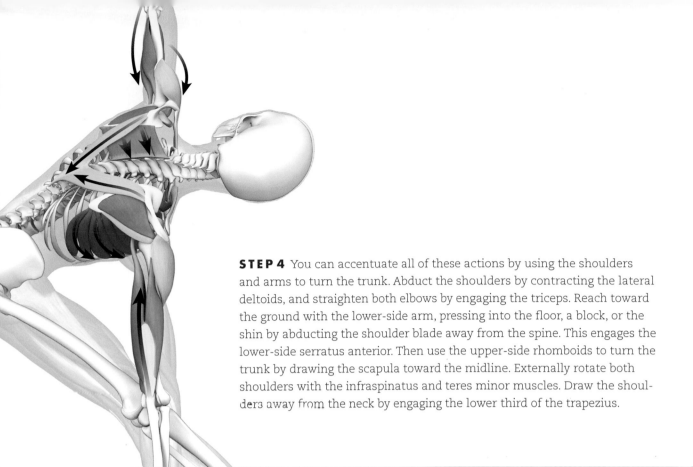

STEP 4 You can accentuate all of these actions by using the shoulders and arms to turn the trunk. Abduct the shoulders by contracting the lateral deltoids, and straighten both elbows by engaging the triceps. Reach toward the ground with the lower-side arm, pressing into the floor, a block, or the shin by abducting the shoulder blade away from the spine. This engages the lower-side serratus anterior. Then use the upper-side rhomboids to turn the trunk by drawing the scapula toward the midline. Externally rotate both shoulders with the infraspinatus and teres minor muscles. Draw the shoulders away from the neck by engaging the lower third of the trapezius.

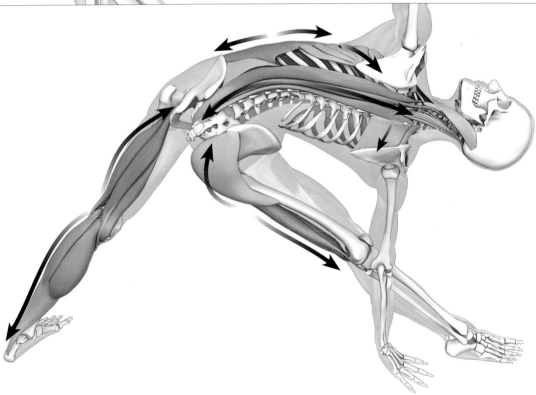

SUMMARY Note how the antagonists of the muscles you have been activating are stretching. The front-leg hamstrings and gluteus maximus are the focal point of the stretch in Utthita Trikonasana, with the upper-side back and abdominals also stretching. The back-leg gastrocnemius and soleus muscles are stretched by dorsiflexion and internal rotation of the foot. Reaching down with the lower-side arm lengthens the rhomboids on this side, and drawing the upper-side scapula toward the midline lengthens the corresponding serratus anterior.

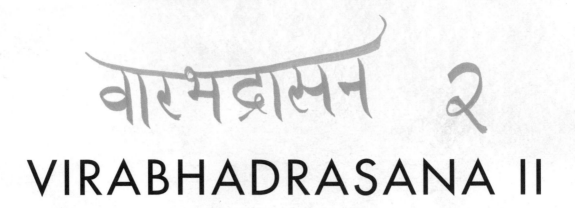

VIRABHADRASANA II

WARRIOR II POSE

THIS POSE EMBODIES THE SPIRIT OF A WARRIOR AND CONVEYS READINESS, stability, and courage. I place Warrior II after Trikonasana because it flows better bio-mechanically, according to the position of the pelvis. This creates continuity in the practice. In both Trikonasana and Warrior II, the pelvis faces relatively forward. In Warriors I and III, it turns toward the front leg. The sequence used in this book illustrates a logical biomechanical progression: for example, readiness (Warrior II), preparing to launch (Warrior I), and launching forward (Warrior III). Each of the warrior poses contains elements of simultaneous movement forward and backward, as well as ascent and descent. These potential movements impart a sense of anticipation of launching energetically forward. The focus of Warrior II is to strengthen the front leg while opening the front of the pelvis and the chest. There can be a tendency to allow the chest to collapse and shift forward. Counteract this by straightening the arms and expanding the chest, expressing the inner strength and confidence that is cultivated in the pose. Build your foundation by planting the back heel firmly on the floor and extending the back arm away from the body. These actions anchor the body against the forward momentum of the pose and bring stability to the posture. If the muscles of the thigh become fatigued, partially straighten the front knee for a moment or two, and then return to the full pose. Tilt the head back slightly and gaze forward.

BASIC JOINT POSITIONS

- The back foot rotates inward 30 degrees and supinates.
- The back knee extends.
- The back hip extends and externally rotates.
- The front hip and knee flex to 90 degrees.
- Both shoulders abduct and externally rotate.
- The elbows extend.
- The forearms pronate.
- The cervical spine rotates to turn the head.

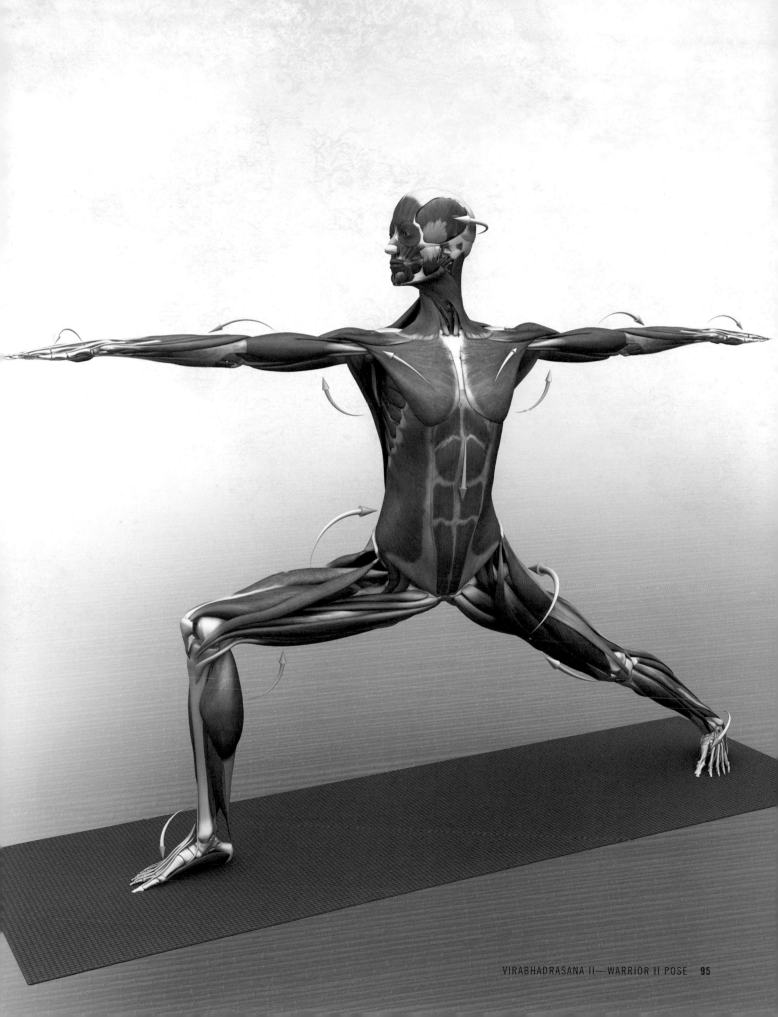

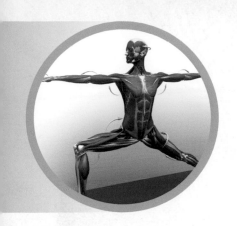

Virabhadrasana II Preparation

Begin by flexing the hip and knee of the front leg. Then place the elbow on the thigh and press down (as with Trikonasana). This action awakens the hip flexors, including the psoas. With the forward hip flexed, engage the muscles of the rear-leg buttocks and lower back to lift the torso and open the chest. In the beginning, you may wish to spend some time conditioning the thigh muscles to maintain the pose. Do this by partially flexing the front knee. Take care to maintain the front hip, thigh, and lower leg in alignment at all times, so that the knee does not drift inward or outward but remains positioned over the ankle. Shift your focus around the body in the pose. For example, if you straighten the knee to rest the thigh of the front leg, remain focused on opening the chest and anchoring the back heel to the floor.

You can also use a folding chair as a prop to experience expanding the chest (thorax) in this pose. Press down with the hands to lift the ribcage as you bend the forward knee into Virabhadrasana II. This activates the latissimus dorsi and lower trapezius as well as the rhomboids. Then raise the arms into the full pose while maintaining the lift of the chest.

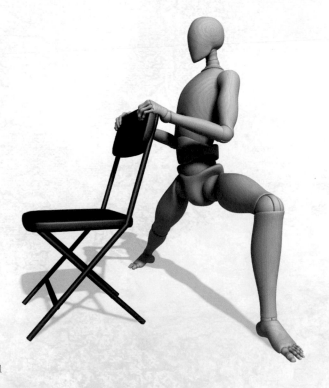

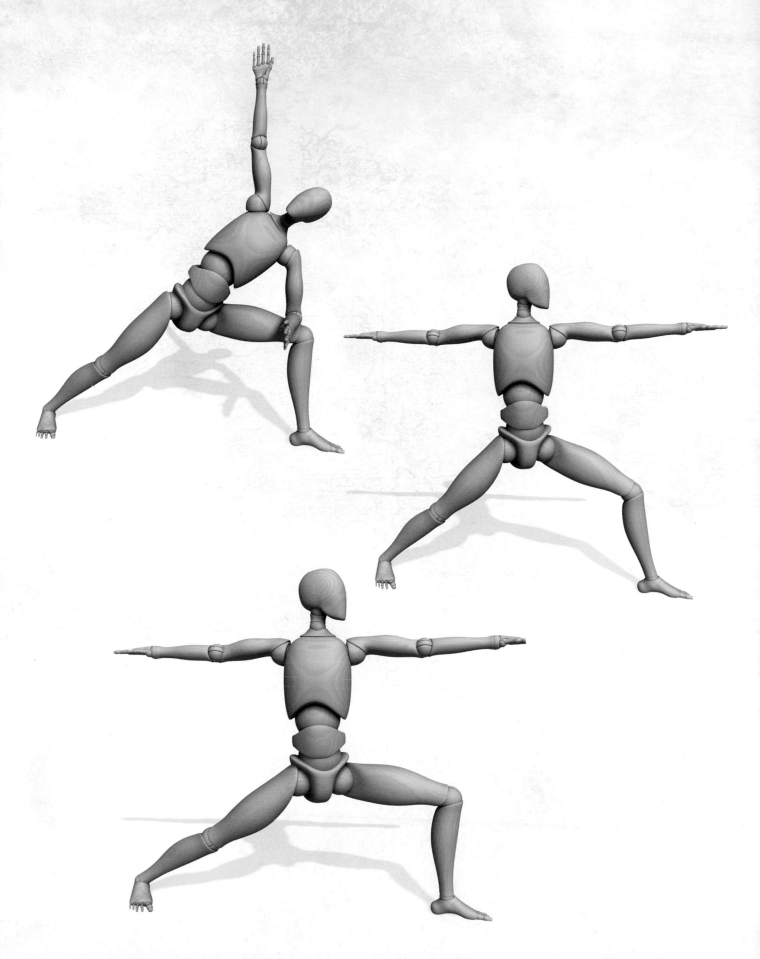

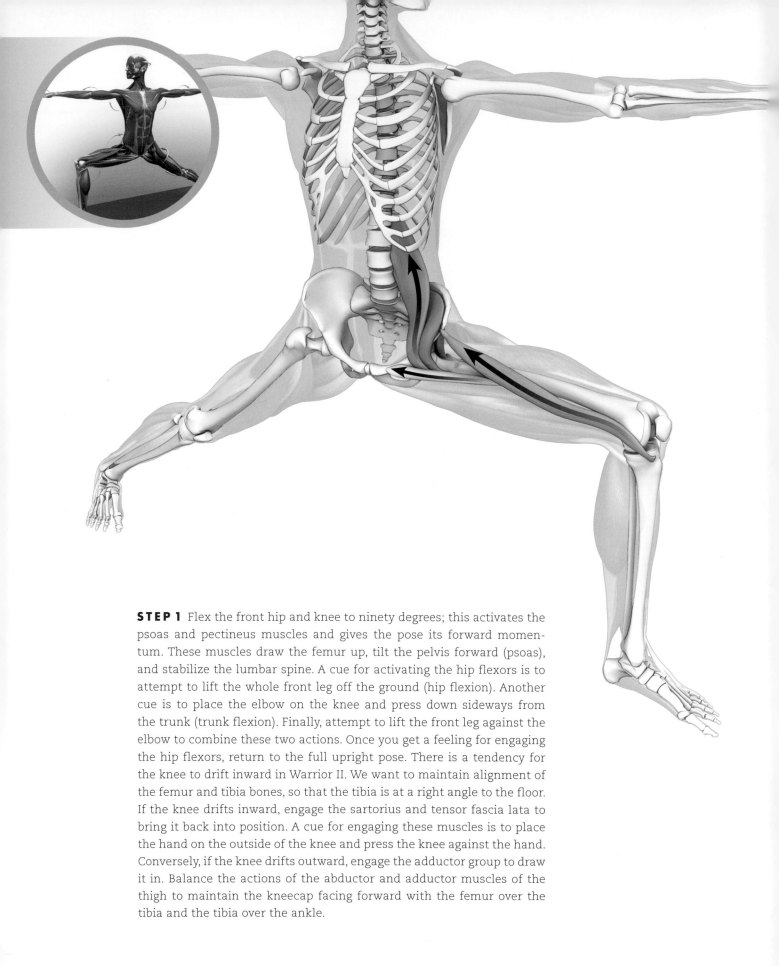

STEP 1 Flex the front hip and knee to ninety degrees; this activates the psoas and pectineus muscles and gives the pose its forward momentum. These muscles draw the femur up, tilt the pelvis forward (psoas), and stabilize the lumbar spine. A cue for activating the hip flexors is to attempt to lift the whole front leg off the ground (hip flexion). Another cue is to place the elbow on the knee and press down sideways from the trunk (trunk flexion). Finally, attempt to lift the front leg against the elbow to combine these two actions. Once you get a feeling for engaging the hip flexors, return to the full upright pose. There is a tendency for the knee to drift inward in Warrior II. We want to maintain alignment of the femur and tibia bones, so that the tibia is at a right angle to the floor. If the knee drifts inward, engage the sartorius and tensor fascia lata to bring it back into position. A cue for engaging these muscles is to place the hand on the outside of the knee and press the knee against the hand. Conversely, if the knee drifts outward, engage the adductor group to draw it in. Balance the actions of the abductor and adductor muscles of the thigh to maintain the kneecap facing forward with the femur over the tibia and the tibia over the ankle.

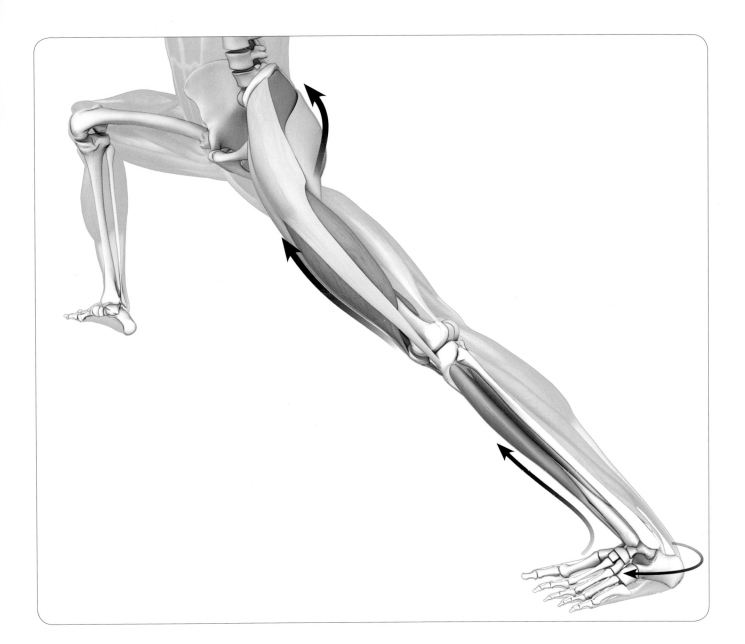

STEP 2 The forward movement created by flexing the front hip and knee is balanced by a line of action through the back leg and heel that anchors the foot to the floor. Activate the tibialis anterior and posterior to dorsiflex and invert the back foot. Then press the outer heel into the mat and activate the quadriceps to straighten the knee. Contract the gluteus medius by attempting to drag the rear foot away from the front, abducting the femur. Squeeze the buttocks and tuck the tailbone to engage the gluteus maximus; this extends the femur. The gluteus maximus also externally rotates the hip, opening the front of the pelvis. Finally, stabilize the back hip by balancing the external rotation created by the gluteus maximus with internal rotation of the thigh. The tensor fascia lata creates this internal rotation in addition to synergizing the quadriceps and stabilizing the back knee.

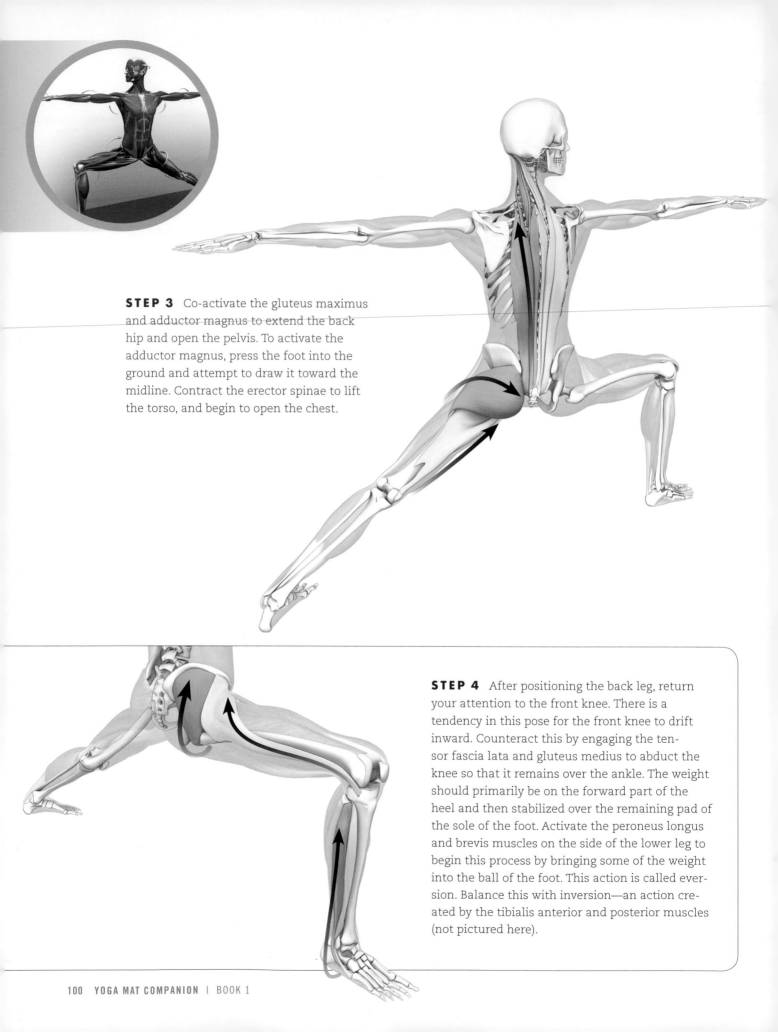

STEP 3 Co-activate the gluteus maximus and adductor magnus to extend the back hip and open the pelvis. To activate the adductor magnus, press the foot into the ground and attempt to draw it toward the midline. Contract the erector spinae to lift the torso, and begin to open the chest.

STEP 4 After positioning the back leg, return your attention to the front knee. There is a tendency in this pose for the front knee to drift inward. Counteract this by engaging the tensor fascia lata and gluteus medius to abduct the knee so that it remains over the ankle. The weight should primarily be on the forward part of the heel and then stabilized over the remaining pad of the sole of the foot. Activate the peroneus longus and brevis muscles on the side of the lower leg to begin this process by bringing some of the weight into the ball of the foot. This action is called eversion. Balance this with inversion—an action created by the tibialis anterior and posterior muscles (not pictured here).

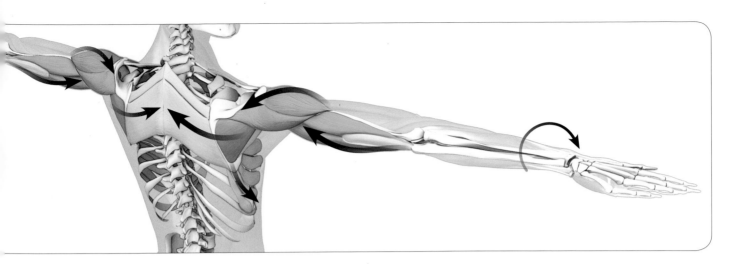

▲ **STEP 5** The shoulders and arms complete the pose. Engage the lateral and posterior deltoids to lift the arms, and then use the infraspinatus and teres minor muscles to externally rotate the upper arm bones at the shoulders. Turn the palms to face down (pronation), using the pronators teres and quadratus. Observe how combining external rotation of the shoulders with pronation of the forearms creates a helical effect up and down the arms, stabilizing them. Contract the rhomboids to draw the scapulae toward the spine while engaging the serratus anterior to spread the arms apart. Co-activation of these muscles stabilizes the shoulder blades and opens the chest. Sculpt this shape by engaging the forward-arm rhomboids and back-arm serratus anterior. Contract the triceps to straighten the elbows. The long head of the triceps also aids in drawing the scapulae away from the midline, broadening the shoulders.

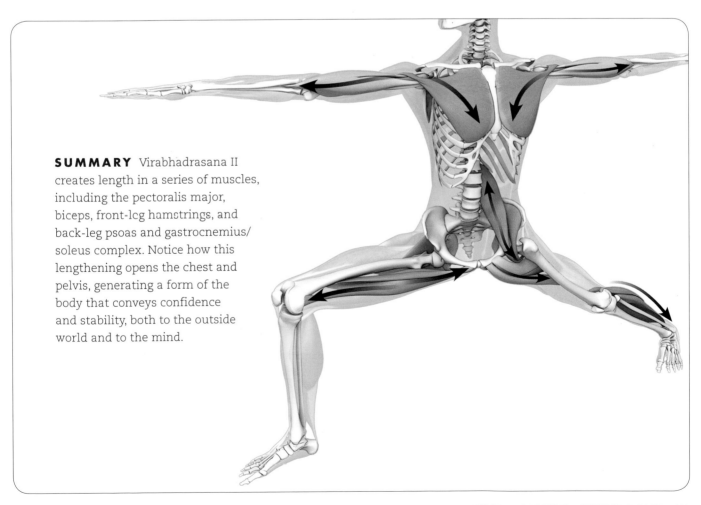

SUMMARY Virabhadrasana II creates length in a series of muscles, including the pectoralis major, biceps, front-leg hamstrings, and back-leg psoas and gastrocnemius/soleus complex. Notice how this lengthening opens the chest and pelvis, generating a form of the body that conveys confidence and stability, both to the outside world and to the mind.

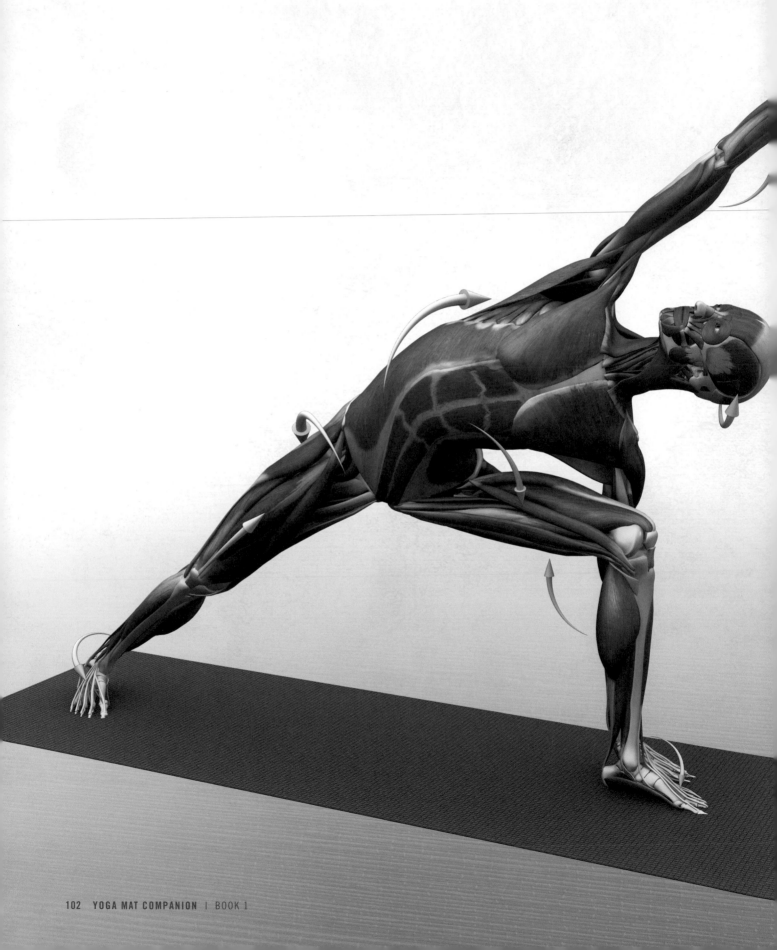

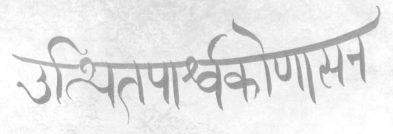

UTTHITA PARSVAKONASANA

EXTENDED LATERAL ANGLE POSE

THIS POSE REPRESENTS A NATURAL PROGRESSION FROM VIRABHADRASANA II—
another example of continuity between poses. Imagine that in Warrior II you are taking
an exaggerated step in preparation to throw a spear. Utthita Parsvakonasana would be the
"follow through" of throwing the spear. We go from an erect trunk in Warrior II to one that
is laterally flexing in this pose. The back arm moves from extending away from the body in
Warrior II to stretching over the head in Utthita Parsvakonasana. Combining the action of
the shoulder and arm with anchoring the back foot into the ground creates a stretch of the
entire upper side of the body. Turn the back foot in and the front foot out ninety degrees.
Straighten the back knee and externally rotate the hip. Flex the torso over the front thigh
and rotate the chest upward from the abdomen. This causes the lower side of the body to
shrink and the upper side to stretch. Look at how the shoulders and pelvis tilt in opposite
directions, communicating with each other through the spine. Press the front foot into the
floor with the weight starting at the posterior heel and spreading across the ball of the foot
and toe mounds. Turn the face slightly upward and tilt the head back.

Remember that the underlying story of this pose is in the breath. Use the accessory
muscles of breathing to open the chest and deepen your inhalations while relaxing into
the exhalations. Turning the body activates the abdominal muscles, which work in con-
junction with the internal intercostals and the elastic recoil of the lungs to aid in exhalation. Remember to ease in and out of the breath to create a sound like waves on a beach.
Use ujjayi breathing.

BASIC JOINT POSITIONS

- The back foot turns in 30 degrees and supinates.
- The front foot turns out 90 degrees.
- The back knee extends.
- The back hip extends and externally rotates.
- The trunk laterally flexes and rotates up.

- The lower-side shoulder abducts and the elbow extends.
- The upper-side arm abducts and flexes overhead, with the elbow extending.
- The upper-side forearm pronates.
- The cervical spine rotates the head to face upward with the neck slightly extended.

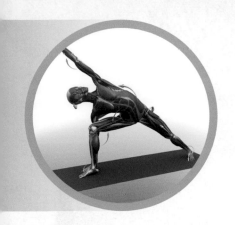

Utthita Parsvakonasana
Preparation

The staging I use in this pose involves isolating and activating the psoas first. Begin by leaning back slightly, raising the arm to stretch the front of the body. Then, place the elbow onto the thigh and press down with the torso, as shown. Contract the back-leg buttocks and feel how this co-contraction of the front-leg psoas and back-leg gluteus maximus stabilizes the pelvis. Straighten the back knee to press the heel into the floor. Extend the arm down and place the hand onto a block or on the floor. Press into the block with the weight of the torso to re-engage the psoas (flexing the trunk). Finally, turn the chest upward and extend from the tips of the fingers to the back heel.

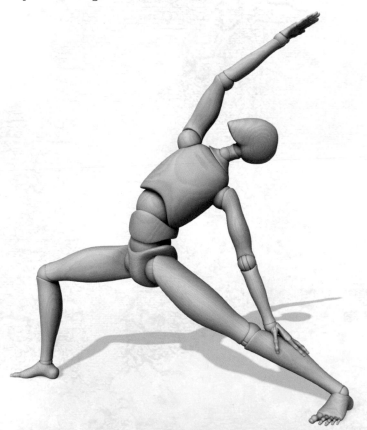

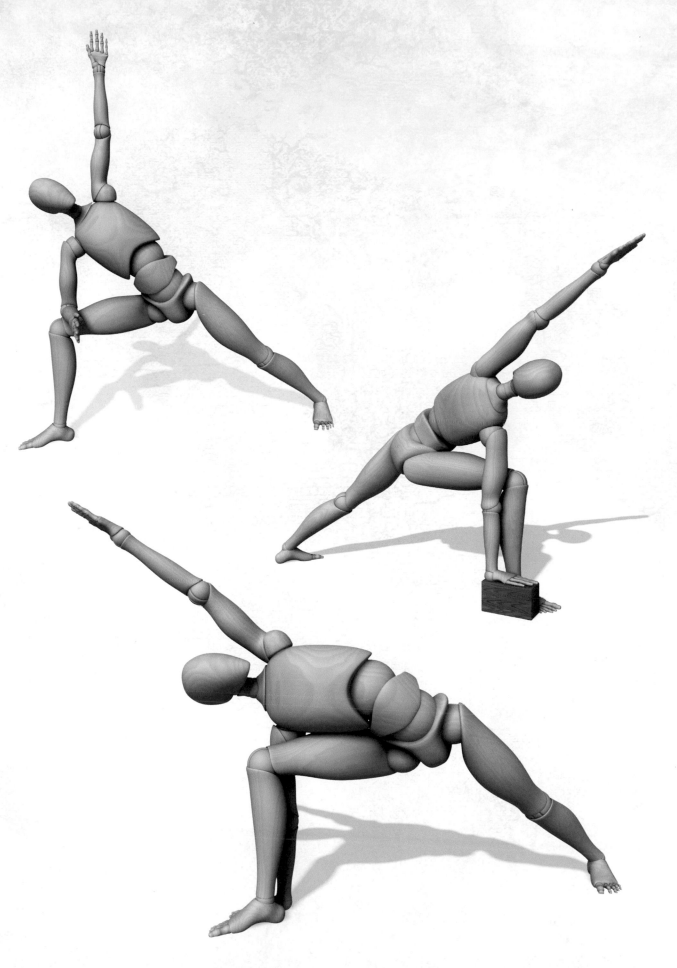

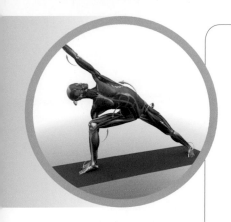

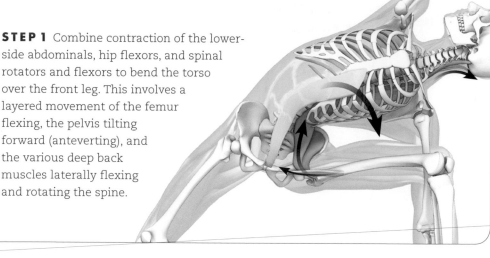

STEP 1 Combine contraction of the lower-side abdominals, hip flexors, and spinal rotators and flexors to bend the torso over the front leg. This involves a layered movement of the femur flexing, the pelvis tilting forward (anteverting), and the various deep back muscles laterally flexing and rotating the spine.

STEP 2 Anchor the back foot into the floor by contracting the tibialis posterior to turn the foot inward (inversion). Then try to draw the top of the foot toward the shin by engaging the tibialis anterior muscle. This presses the heel down. Straighten the knee by activating the quadriceps and its synergist, the tensor fascia lata. Co-activate the gluteus medius and adductor magnus to stabilize the femur in the hip socket. The cue for this is to attempt to drag the back foot away from the front, while pressing the sole of the foot into the floor.

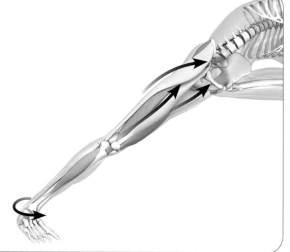

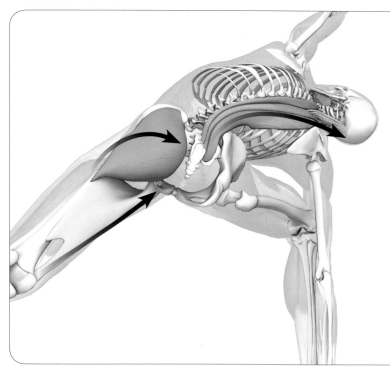

STEP 3 This image shows a combination of muscles that can be used concurrently to extend the back body and open the front body. The gluteus maximus forms the cornerstone, extending and externally rotating the back femur. The adductor magnus synergizes this extension. The cue for engaging these muscles together is to press the sole of the back foot into the floor and drag it toward the back side of the mat. The lower-side erector spinae both flexes the trunk and opens the chest forward and upward. The cue for this action is to arch the lower-side back.

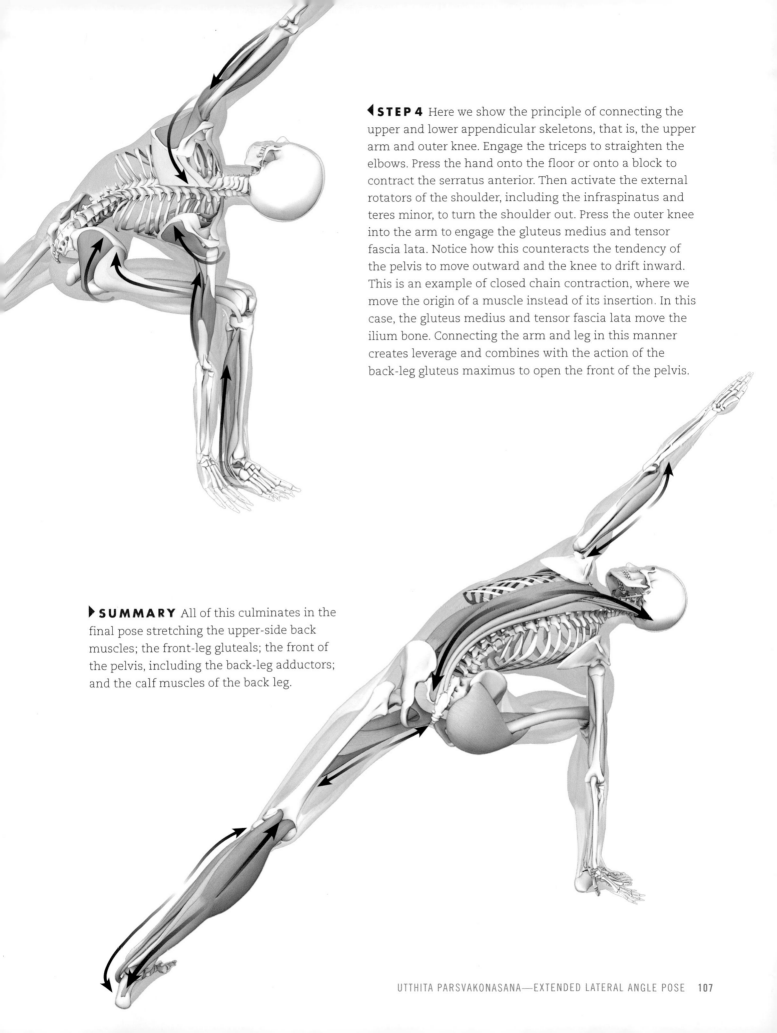

◀ STEP 4 Here we show the principle of connecting the upper and lower appendicular skeletons, that is, the upper arm and outer knee. Engage the triceps to straighten the elbows. Press the hand onto the floor or onto a block to contract the serratus anterior. Then activate the external rotators of the shoulder, including the infraspinatus and teres minor, to turn the shoulder out. Press the outer knee into the arm to engage the gluteus medius and tensor fascia lata. Notice how this counteracts the tendency of the pelvis to move outward and the knee to drift inward. This is an example of closed chain contraction, where we move the origin of a muscle instead of its insertion. In this case, the gluteus medius and tensor fascia lata move the ilium bone. Connecting the arm and leg in this manner creates leverage and combines with the action of the back-leg gluteus maximus to open the front of the pelvis.

▶ SUMMARY All of this culminates in the final pose stretching the upper-side back muscles; the front-leg gluteals; the front of the pelvis, including the back-leg adductors; and the calf muscles of the back leg.

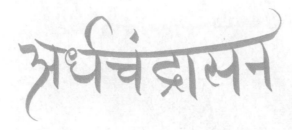

ARDHA CHANDRASANA

HALF-MOON POSE

THE MAIN STORY OR THE PRIMARY FOCUS OF ARDHA CHANDRASANA IS AN INTENSE stretch of the hamstring, gluteal, and gastrocnemius muscles on the back of the standing leg. A subplot is the balancing act that takes place in the pose. The actions of maintaining our balance and stretching the muscles on the back of the standing leg are interconnected. For example, contracting the quadriceps and hip flexors of the standing leg helps to maintain balance but also signals the muscles at the back of the leg that are stretching, the hamstrings and gluteals, to relax through the physiological process of reciprocal inhibition. Ardha Chandrasana is a natural progression from the previous two postures (Virabhadrasana II and Utthita Parsvakonasana), projecting the body forward into a balancing pose. Combining the poses in this manner creates synergy and continuity within the practice.

Use the principle of triangulation to locate the focal point in Half-Moon. Triangulation does not necessarily refer to a geometric triangle, but rather a conceptual one, wherein the actions of two structures work together to affect a third. In Ardha Chandrasana, flexing the trunk tilts the pelvis forward and draws the origin (ischial tuberosity) of the standing-leg hamstrings up; this forms one corner of the triangle. Straightening the standing leg takes the insertion of these same muscles in the other direction, forming another corner of the triangle. These two actions combine to lengthen (stretch) the standing-leg hamstrings, creating an apex for our conceptual triangle.

Now, what about the subplot in this pose, the balancing act? How can we use basic principles of physics to assist in the asana? First, if you start to lose balance, you can regain stability by bending the standing knee. Slightly lower the raised leg for additional stability. Both of these actions lower the center of gravity and make it easier to balance. Once you regain stability, engage the quadriceps to straighten the knee while keeping the hip flexed over the thigh. Use the raised leg like a tight-rope walker uses a pole. That is, if you start to fall back, shift the raised leg forward; if you start to fall forward, shift the leg back. The soundtrack of the pose is the breath; focus on your breathing to improve your balance.

BASIC JOINT POSITIONS

- The standing hip flexes.
- Both knees extend.
- The raised hip externally rotates.

- The shoulders abduct.
- The cervical spine rotates the head to face upward or remains neutral.

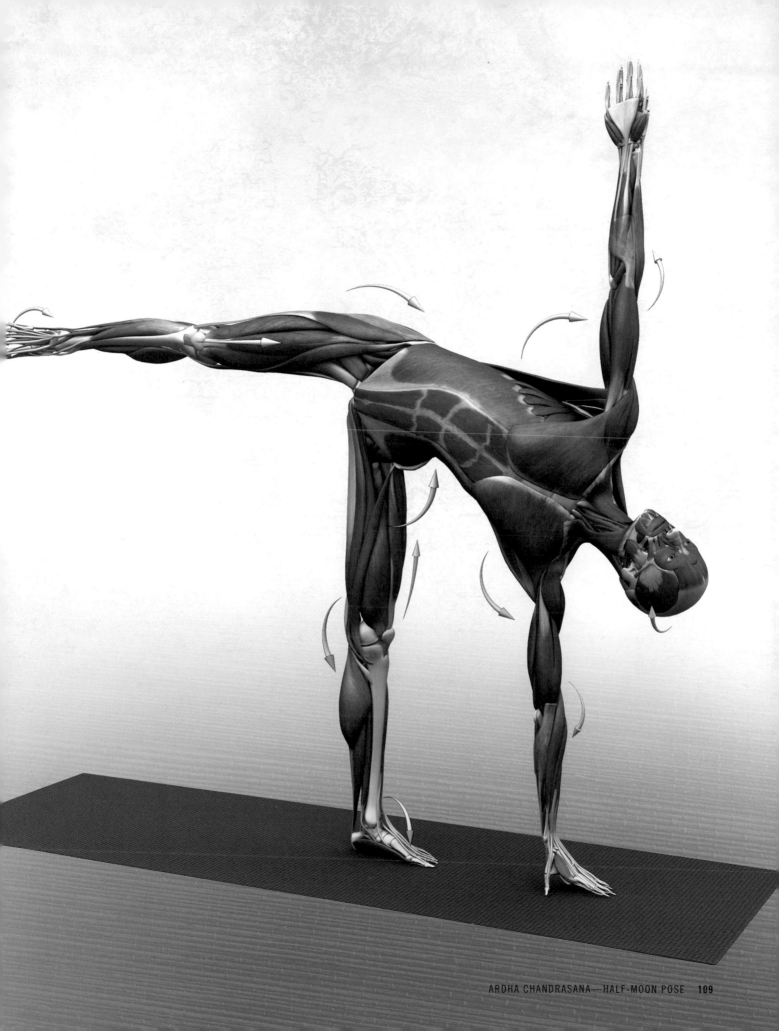

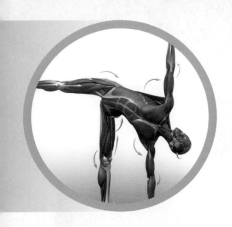

Ardha Chandrasana Preparation

To activate the psoas muscle, bend forward and place the elbow on the knee and press down with the torso. Alternatively, come straight into a shallow Trikonasana. Next, bend the standing leg and step the back foot forward about one foot; at the same time, place the hand about twelve inches in front and to the outside of the standing leg.

Lean the weight forward onto the hand and begin to lift the straight back leg, like a teeter totter. Maintain the standing leg bent and align the pelvis over the ankle. Finally, lift the torso by activating the quadriceps to straighten the standing leg (extending the knee) in an action similar to a hydraulic lift. Use the upper arm for balance and as a tool to lever the chest open.

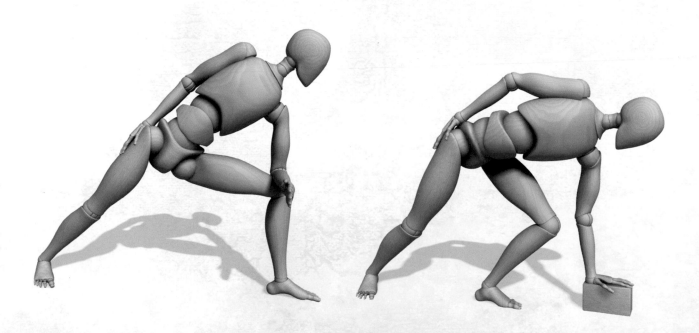

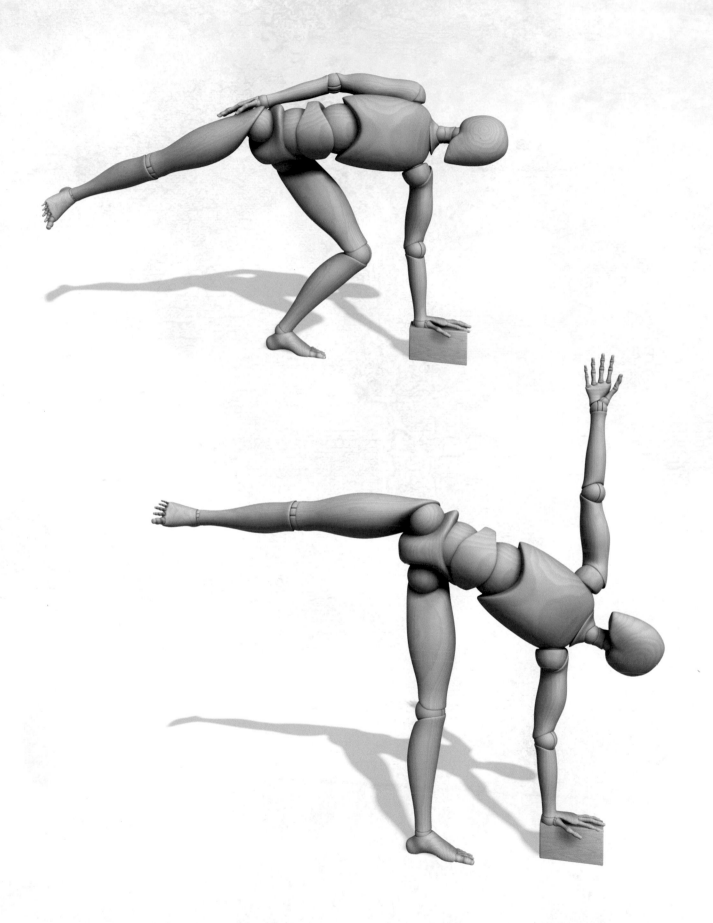

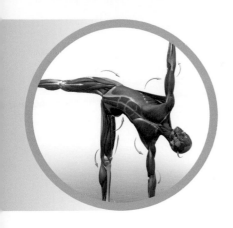

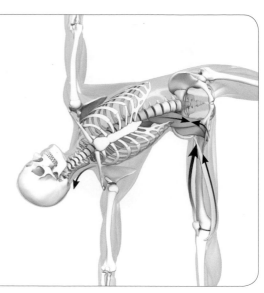

STEP 1 Laterally flex the trunk by engaging the oblique abdominals, the deep back muscles, and the hip flexors. Use the image here to aid in visualizing these muscles contracting. Notice how the rectus femoris and sartorius muscles cross the pelvis and hip, making them synergistic hip flexors. You can engage the rectus femoris by lifting the kneecap toward the pelvis.

STEP 2 Lift the back leg using the hip abductors—the gluteus medius, gluteus minimus, and tensor fascia lata. One of your goals is to have the kneecap of the raised leg facing directly forward. If it is facing upward, internally rotate the thigh bone by engaging the gluteus medius and tensor fascia lata. Activate the quadriceps to straighten the knee. Evert the foot by contracting the muscles on the outside of the lower leg, the peroneus longus and brevis. This action opens the sole of the foot, stimulating the minor chakras in this region.

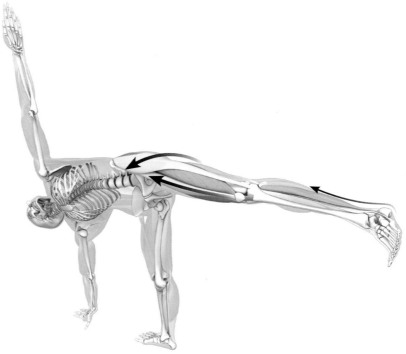

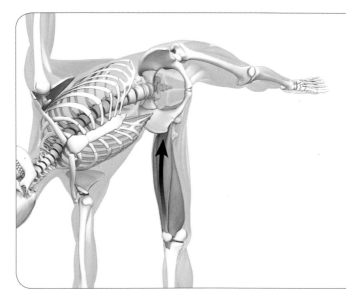

STEP 3 Firmly contract the quadriceps of the standing leg. This straightens the knee, lifting the pelvis and trunk upward. Extending the knee moves the insertion of the hamstrings on the lower leg farther away from their origin on the ischial tuberosity. Contracting the quadriceps initiates reciprocal inhibition of the hamstrings, causing them to safely relax into the stretch.

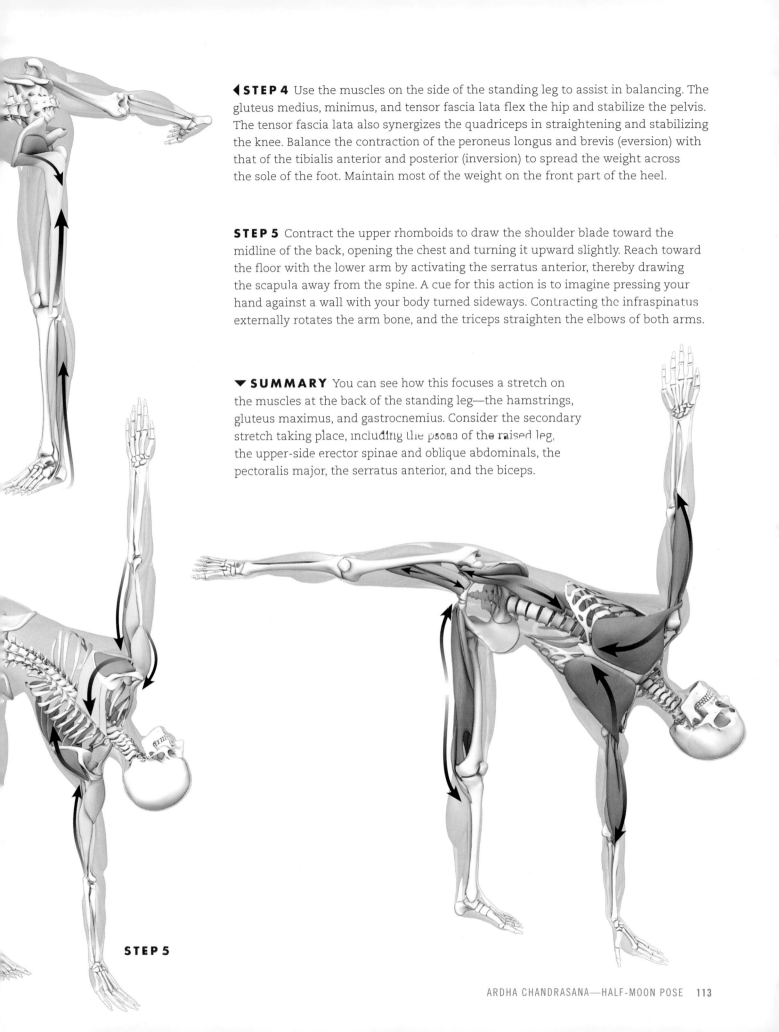

◀ STEP 4 Use the muscles on the side of the standing leg to assist in balancing. The gluteus medius, minimus, and tensor fascia lata flex the hip and stabilize the pelvis. The tensor fascia lata also synergizes the quadriceps in straightening and stabilizing the knee. Balance the contraction of the peroneus longus and brevis (eversion) with that of the tibialis anterior and posterior (inversion) to spread the weight across the sole of the foot. Maintain most of the weight on the front part of the heel.

STEP 5 Contract the upper rhomboids to draw the shoulder blade toward the midline of the back, opening the chest and turning it upward slightly. Reach toward the floor with the lower arm by activating the serratus anterior, thereby drawing the scapula away from the spine. A cue for this action is to imagine pressing your hand against a wall with your body turned sideways. Contracting the infraspinatus externally rotates the arm bone, and the triceps straighten the elbows of both arms.

▼ SUMMARY You can see how this focuses a stretch on the muscles at the back of the standing leg—the hamstrings, gluteus maximus, and gastrocnemius. Consider the secondary stretch taking place, including the psoas of the raised leg, the upper-side erector spinae and oblique abdominals, the pectoralis major, the serratus anterior, and the biceps.

STEP 5

पार्श्वोत्तानासन

PARSVOTTANASANA

INTENSE SIDE-STRETCH POSE

IN PARSVOTTANASANA, THE PELVIS ROTATES TO FACE THE FRONT LEG. I PLACE THIS POSE after Ardha Chandrasana to create continuity in the sequence. Later in the practice we rotate the pelvis further, so that this type of pose fits naturally in a sequence that moves from the pelvis facing forward, to turning the pelvis to face the front leg, to rotating into a twisting pose such as Parivrtta Trikonasana. Turning the pelvis changes the orientation of the muscle fibers in the back-leg gluteals and front-leg hip flexors, activating the muscle from every direction. This illustrates how designing your yoga practice to have continuity yet change awakens muscle groups efficiently, making the whole of the practice greater than the sum of its parts.

The focal point of the stretch in Parsvottanasana is the front-leg hamstrings. Remember to firmly engage the quadriceps and hip flexors to stimulate reciprocal inhibition of the hamstrings; observe how engaging these muscles changes the sensation of the stretch. A subplot of this pose is the stretch of the back-leg hamstrings and gastrocnemius. The position of the pelvis, back hip, and back foot create a unique opportunity to stretch these muscles. Augment this stretch by attempting to drag the back foot away from the front foot on the mat, opening the back of the knee.

The classical version of Parsvottanasana has the hands in prayer position (namasté) on the back. This is one example of the ancient yogis devising a way to stretch some of the more hidden and difficult-to-access muscles—the external rotators of the shoulders, including the infraspinatus and teres minor, as well as elements of the deltoids and other muscles. Be careful not to put undue pressure on the extended wrists in this pose.

BASIC JOINT POSITIONS

- The back foot rotates inward 30 degrees and supinates.
- The front foot rotates out 90 degrees.
- The trunk flexes.
- The front hip flexes and externally rotates.

- The back hip internally rotates.
- The knees extend.
- The shoulders internally rotate.
- The wrists extend.
- The cervical spine flexes slightly.

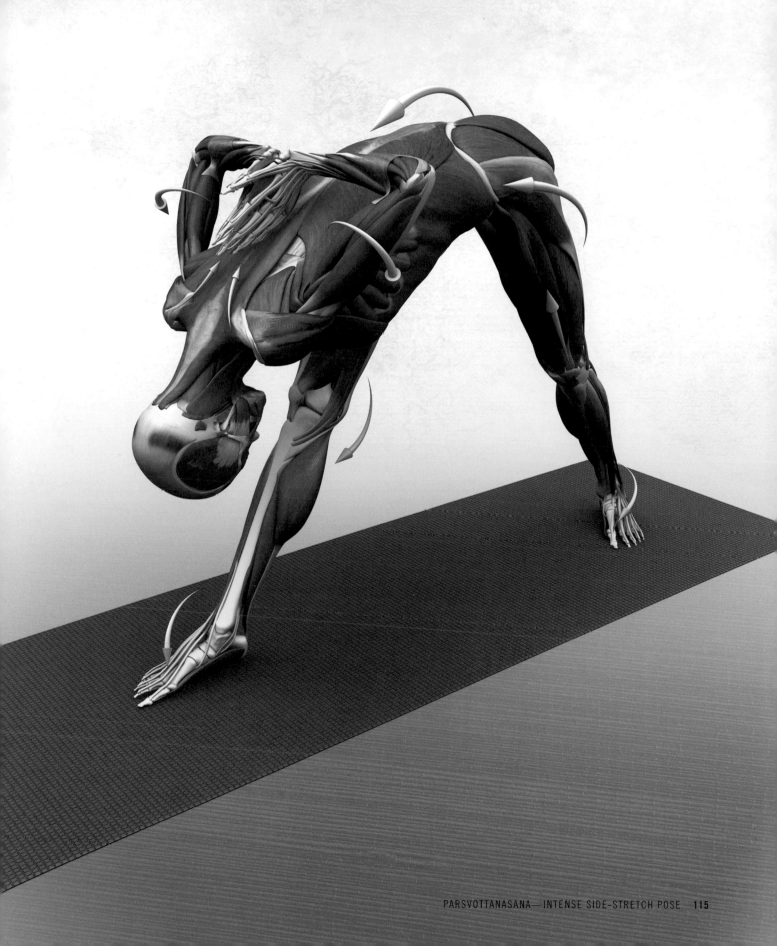

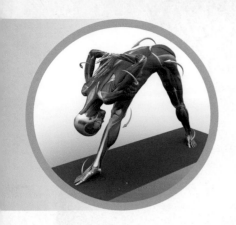

Parsvottanasana Preparation

Begin by positioning the hands in reverse namasté while standing in Tadasana or with the feet apart. Do not force your hands into this position, as you can injure your wrists (do not let anyone else force your hands into this position either). Roll the shoulders forward to release the external rotators. Take advantage of this release and move your hands higher up the back; then roll your shoulders back again. If you are unable to comfortably place the hands in reverse namasté, then hold the elbows, forearms, or wrists. Internally rotate the back foot about thirty degrees, with the front foot turned out ninety degrees. Lift the chest with a deep inhalation. Bend the front-leg knee to release the hamstrings, allowing you to bring the torso into contact with or close to the front thigh. If the shoulders are tight, you can also place the hands on either side of the foot, as shown. Squeeze the torso against the thigh to activate the hip and trunk flexors; maintain this position of the trunk, and contract the quadriceps to straighten the knee. If you feel strain at the back of the leg, lift the torso off the thigh. Carefully come out of the pose by maintaining the front femur in alignment with the lower leg. Bend the front knee, and push yourself up by straightening the leg. Use the extensor muscles of the back to lift the chest.

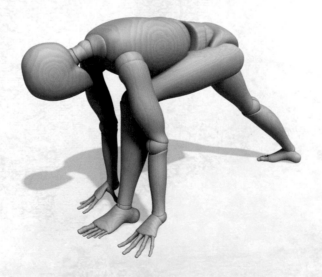

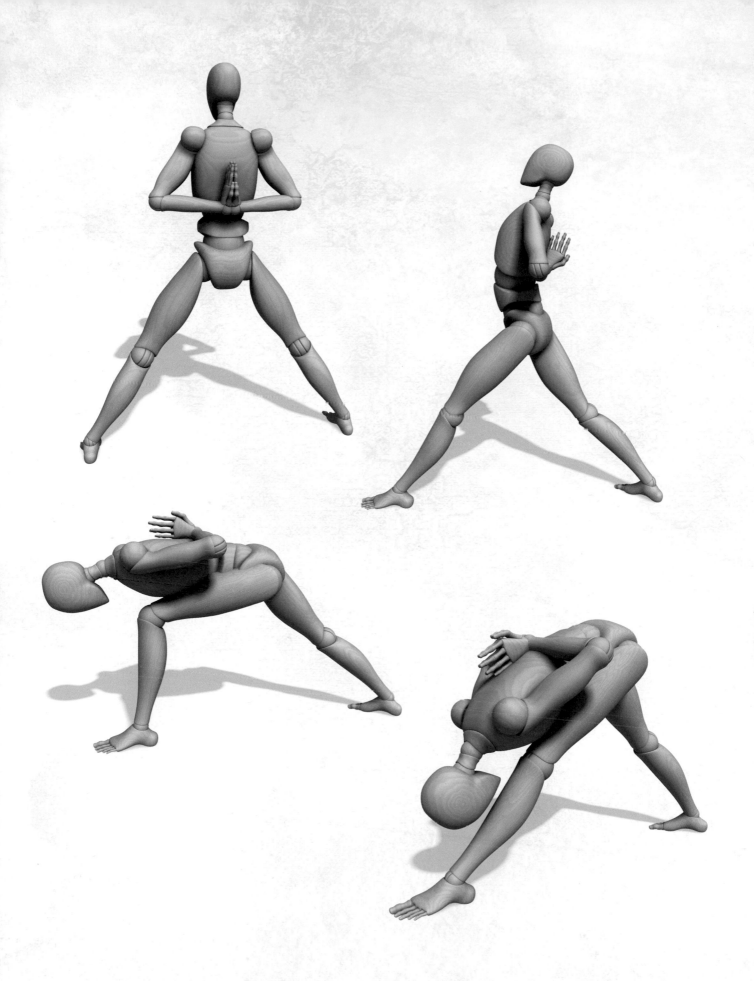

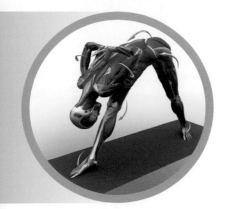

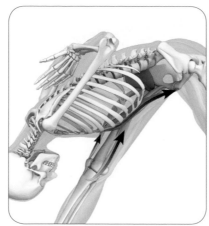

◄STEP 1 Use the hip and trunk flexors to draw the torso over the thigh. The main hip flexor, the psoas, tilts the pelvis forward, lifting the ischial tuberosity (the origin of the hamstrings) up and back. This stretches the front-leg hamstrings. Note that one of the heads of the quadriceps, the rectus femoris muscle, crosses the hip joint. When you engage the quadriceps to straighten the knee, this muscle synergizes the psoas in flexing the hip. Engage the abdominals, including the rectus abdominis, to flex the trunk forward.

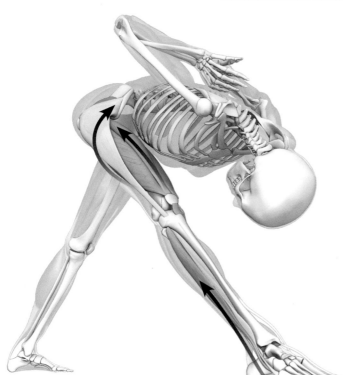

◄STEP 2 Contract the quadriceps to straighten the knee and stretch the hamstrings. Feel how the hamstrings become taut. This is because stretching a muscle causes it to contract—an unconscious reflex that aids to protect the muscle from tearing. You can safely overcome this reflex by engaging the antagonist muscle group, in this case the quadriceps. This stimulates an alternative reflex known as reciprocal inhibition that signals the muscle to relax into the stretch.

There is a tendency to shift the weight onto the outside of the front foot in this pose, inverting the ankle. Counteract this by engaging the peroneus longus and brevis muscles on the outside of the leg to evert the ankle and press the ball of the foot into the mat.

▶STEP 3 Look at the subplot in the back leg. The back knee is straight with the ankle turning in and dorsiflexing. Engage the quadriceps to straighten the knee, the tibialis anterior to dorsiflex the ankle, and the tibialis posterior to invert the foot. This creates reciprocal inhibition of the hamstrings and gastrocnemius/soleus complex, allowing them to relax into the stretch. Augment this stretch by attempting to drag the back foot away from the front. This cue stimulates the back-leg gluteals and adductor magnus to contract. The force of the contraction is transmitted to the back of the knee, further stretching the hamstrings and gastrocnemius/soleus complex.

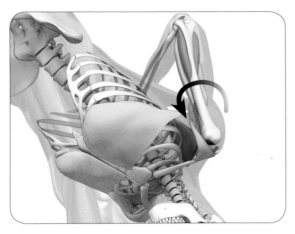 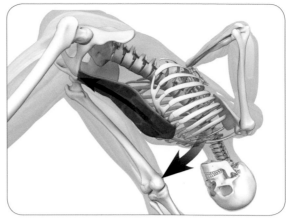

STEP 4 Observe the muscles used to bring the hands into namasté position on the back. The biomechanics of this position stretch the external rotators of the shoulders. Accentuate this stretch by contracting the lower pectoralis major; the cue for this is to roll the shoulders forward, contracting the muscle at the front of the chest. The anterior deltoids, the muscles that lift the arms overhead, also internally rotate the shoulders. Visualize contracting these muscles to accentuate this internal rotation. Similarly, visualize the subscapularis muscles on the insides of the shoulder blades contracting to rotate the shoulders inward. Bend the elbows to engage the biceps, synergizing the subscapularis. Train yourself to engage these muscles even when the arms are behind the back. Activate the rectus abdominis muscle to flex the trunk. Feel how this action increases the stretch of the shoulders.

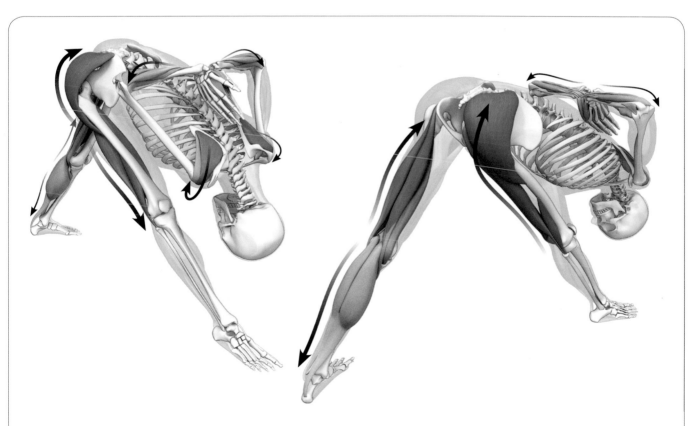

SUMMARY This image gives a view of the muscles that stretch when the upper extremities are in reverse namasté. These include the infraspinatus and teres minor muscles of the rotator cuff and the wrist flexors. Although the front-leg hamstrings and gluteals are the main focus of the pose, you can accentuate the stretch of the back-leg hamstrings and gastrocnemius/soleus complex as described.

वीरभद्रासन २

VIRABHADRASANA I

WARRIOR I POSE

WARRIOR I ILLUSTRATES THE CONCEPT OF CREATING STILLNESS BY BALANCING simultaneous movements in different directions. The front hip flexors and back hip extensors engage to descend and stabilize the pelvis while the chest lifts upward toward the sky. Similarly, the front hip and knee flex to create a sense of forward movement while the back hip and knee extend to constrain the rear foot onto the mat. As a result of these simultaneous movements, the body becomes a storehouse for potential energy, like a sprinter preparing to bolt out of the blocks.

Positioning Warrior I after Parsvottanasana in the standing pose sequence creates a synergistic progression that continues the turn of the pelvis from facing forward in poses such as Trikonasana and Warrior II, to facing toward the front leg in Warrior I. Placing Warrior I after Parsvottanasana balances folding forward (Parsvottanasana) with expanding upward (Warrior I). In Parsvottanasana the torso folds over the leg to create a deep stretch along the back side of the body; Warrior I rises from this position, expanding from the core and extending upward through the chest.

BASIC JOINT POSITIONS

- The back foot turns inward 30 degrees and supinates.
- The front foot turns out 90 degrees.
- The back hip and knee extend.

- The front hip and knee flex.
- The shoulders flex overhead.
- The elbows extend.
- The back extends.
- The cervical spine extends.

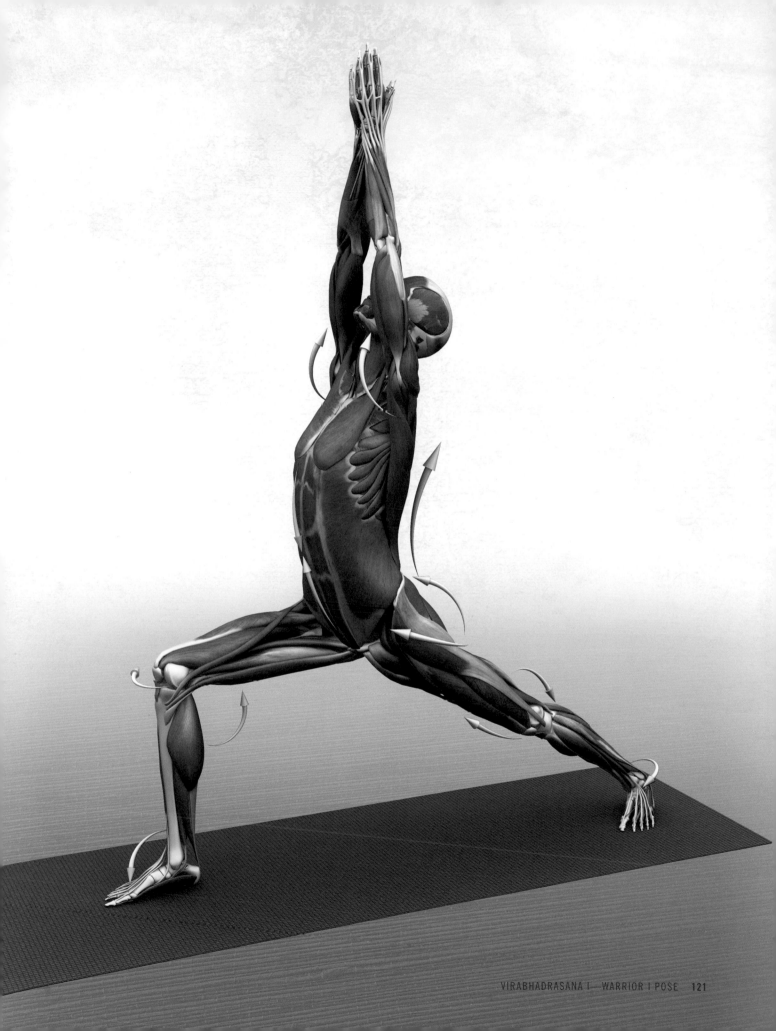

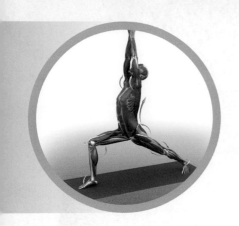

Virabhadrasana I Preparation

Take the general form of the pose by turning the hips toward the front leg. Activate the back-leg buttocks and thigh muscles. Raise the arms and lift the chest. In this position, flex the front hip and knee to ninety degrees (keep the knee aligned over the ankle). In the beginning or when you feel fatigued, lessen the bend in the knee to make the pose easier. Maintain the alignment of the front-leg femur and tibia when you come out of the pose. This aids to protect the knee joint. You can also add a stretch of the front hip extensors to the preparation by using the bent-knee version of Supta Padangusthasana.

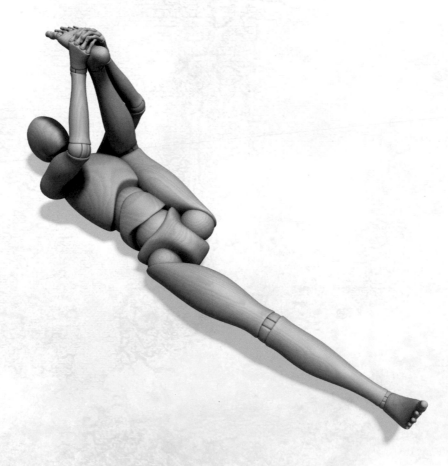

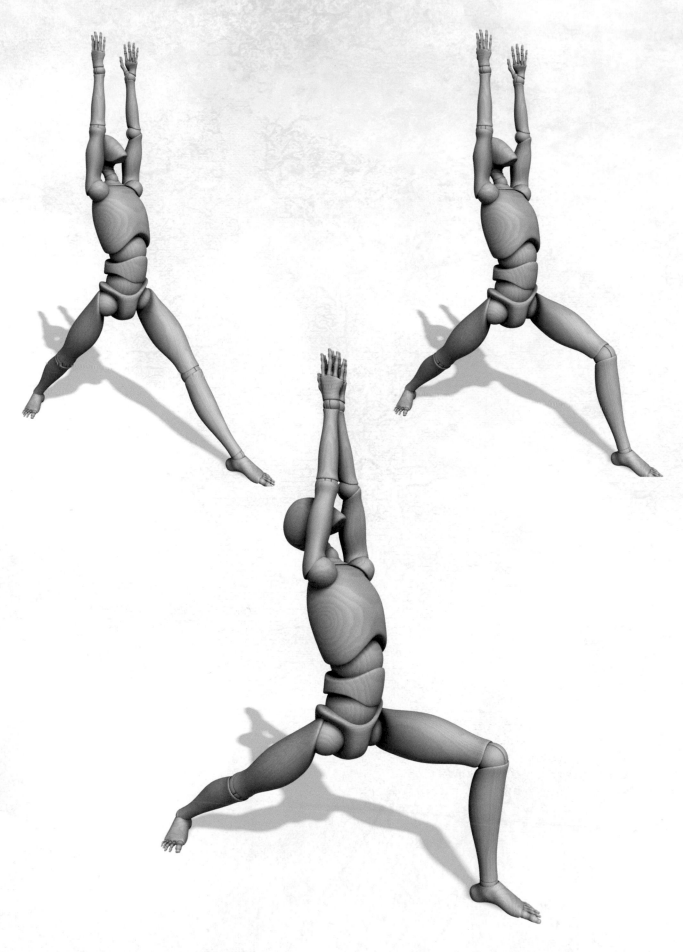

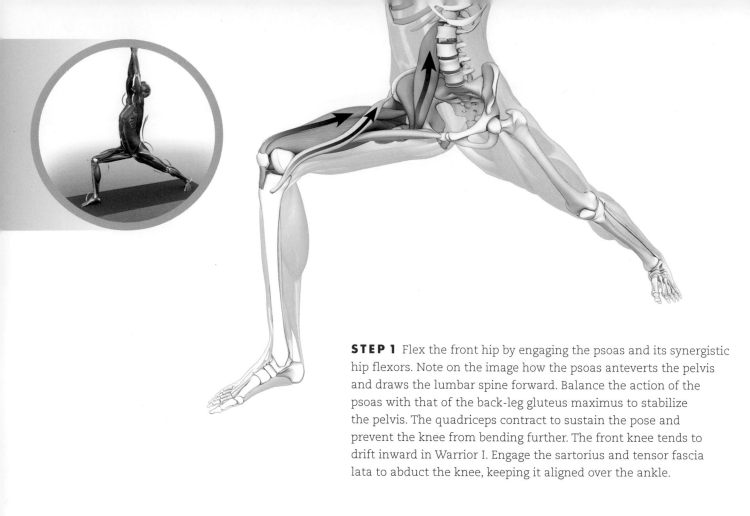

STEP 1 Flex the front hip by engaging the psoas and its synergistic hip flexors. Note on the image how the psoas anteverts the pelvis and draws the lumbar spine forward. Balance the action of the psoas with that of the back-leg gluteus maximus to stabilize the pelvis. The quadriceps contract to sustain the pose and prevent the knee from bending further. The front knee tends to drift inward in Warrior I. Engage the sartorius and tensor fascia lata to abduct the knee, keeping it aligned over the ankle.

STEP 2 The muscles that extend the back of the body create a line of action from the heel to the pelvis and up the spine. These muscles include the tibialis anterior, adductor magnus, gluteus maximus and minimus, quadratus lumborum, and erector spinae. Draw the top of the foot toward the shin to engage the tibialis anterior. Feel how this presses the heel into the floor. Attempt to drag the back foot toward the midline to engage the adductor magnus. Feel how this extends the leg. Engage the gluteus maximus to extend and externally rotate the hip. Visualize the gluteus minimus synergizing this action. Co-contract the buttocks muscles and the muscles of the back, including the quadratus lumborum and erector spinae, to lift the trunk and open the chest. Do this by arching the back while squeezing the buttocks.

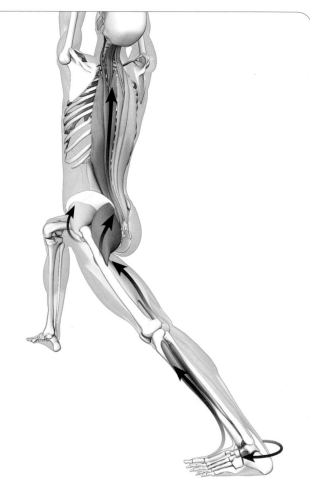

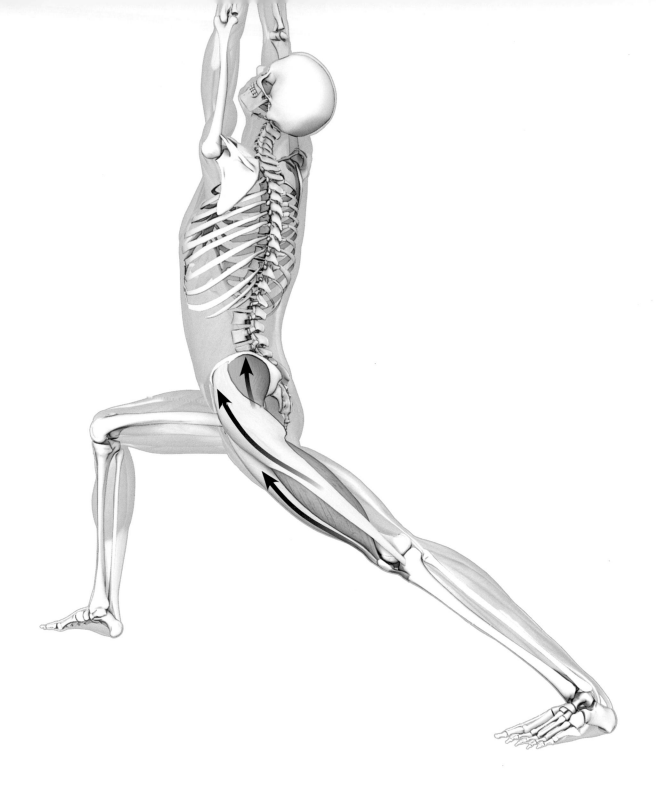

STEP 3 Combine the action of the back-leg tibialis anterior described in Step 2 with that of the quadriceps. Extend the knee while attempting to lift the top of the foot toward the shin, pressing the heel down. Engage the tensor fascia lata to assist the quadriceps and help the gluteus medius turn the entire leg inward. Note that the gluteus maximus (Step 2) not only extends the hip but externally rotates it as well. Engaging the tensor fascia lata and gluteus medius balances the external rotation produced by the gluteus maximus with a force that turns the hip inward. This stabilizes and turns the pelvis forward.

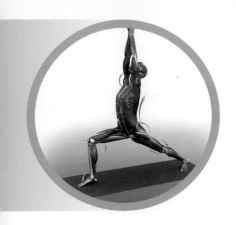

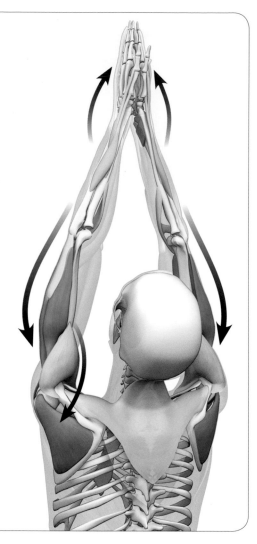

STEP 4 Use the arms and shoulders to lift the upper body and chest away from the pelvis, creating the upward movement in the pose. Contract the trapezius to lift the shoulders, the triceps to straighten the elbows, the deltoids to lift the arms, and the infraspinatus and teres minor muscles to externally rotate the humeri. Press the mounds of the index fingers together to pronate the forearms, using the pronators teres and quadratus. Balance pronation of the forearms by extending and abducting the thumbs. This engages the extensor pollicis longus and abductor pollicis muscles, minor supinators of the forearms. Note that, once the shoulders are lifted, we will relax the upper third of the trapezius and allow the lower third to draw the shoulders away from the ears in a sequential action, as illustrated in Step 5.

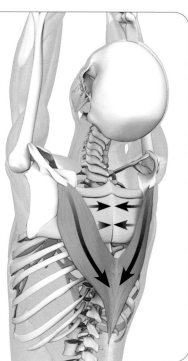

STEP 5 Draw the shoulders down the back by contracting the lower trapezius. Engage the rhomboids to stabilize the shoulder blades toward the midline. These actions combine to draw the shoulders away from the ears and open the chest forward. The rhomboids act to stabilize the shoulder blades and prepare them for closed chain contraction of the pectoralis minor and serratus anterior muscles, as described in Step 6.

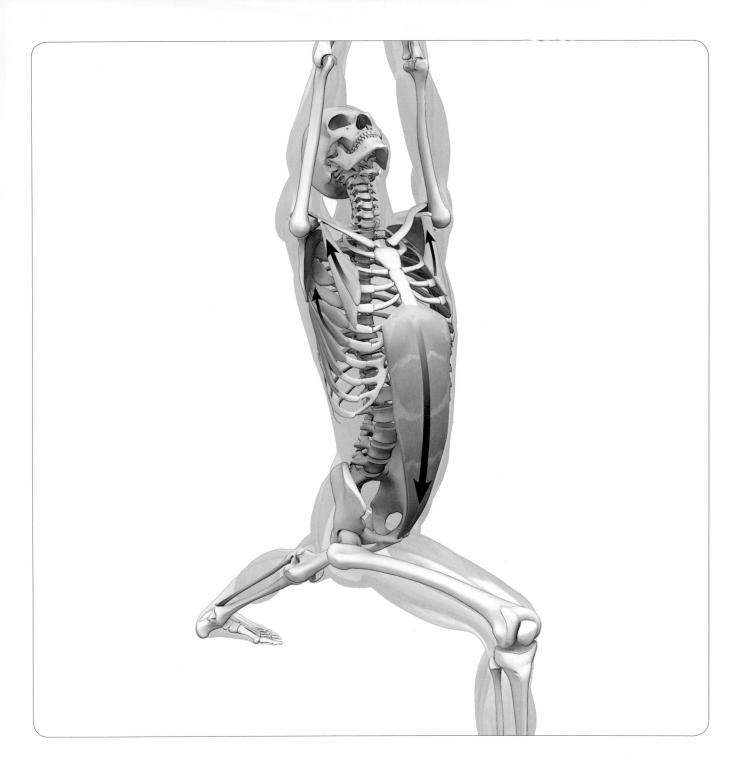

STEP 6 The pectoralis minor and serratus anterior can be used to expand the thorax upward in Virabhadrasana I. This begins with stabilizing the shoulder blades toward the midline, as described in Step 5. It can be difficult and even frustrating to contract these muscles when the arms are overhead. Nevertheless, it can be done and will create more lift and expansion in the chest in this pose. Train yourself to combine these muscle actions in poses such as Tadasana first. Then integrate them into other poses, such as Warrior I.

Engage the rectus abdominis muscle to draw the lower ribs downward and prevent them from bulging forward. Use small actions such as these to put the final touch on a pose.

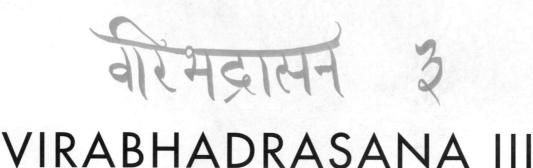

VIRABHADRASANA III

WARRIOR III POSE

WARRIOR III CONVERTS THE POTENTIAL ENERGY STORED IN WARRIOR I INTO movement, projecting the body forward into a balance on the front leg. The main story of the pose is the rotation of the pelvis toward and flexion of the torso over the standing leg. Note how this stretches the back of the standing leg differently than in a pose that has the pelvis facing forward, such as Ardha Chandrasana.

The back story in Warrior III is the balancing act. As with all balancing poses, become aware of your center of gravity and use it to your advantage. Bend the standing leg and/or lower the lifted leg to descend the center of gravity and make the pose more stable. Remember that stability in all of the standing postures, whether balancing on one leg or standing on both, originates from the large muscles of the pelvic core—the psoas and the gluteals. A small movement of the femur at the hip translates into a large movement of the foot, causing you to waver. This is the physics of a lever arm. Similarly, a small movement of the lower trunk translates into a large movement of the shoulders and arms. Once the legs and arms begin to move, it becomes difficult to regain balance. Conversely, stabilizing the pelvis and hip joint prevents the trunk and extremities from wavering.

Another advantage to engaging these core muscles of the pelvis, aside from conferring biomechanical stability, is stimulation of the sensory and motor nerves in the region of the pelvis. Increased activity in these nerves illuminates the first and second chakras. The soundtrack for this balancing act is the breath.

BASIC JOINT POSITIONS

- The standing hip flexes.
- The raised hip extends and internally rotates.
- The knees extend.

- The shoulders flex and the elbows extend.
- The back extends.
- The cervical spine extends slightly.

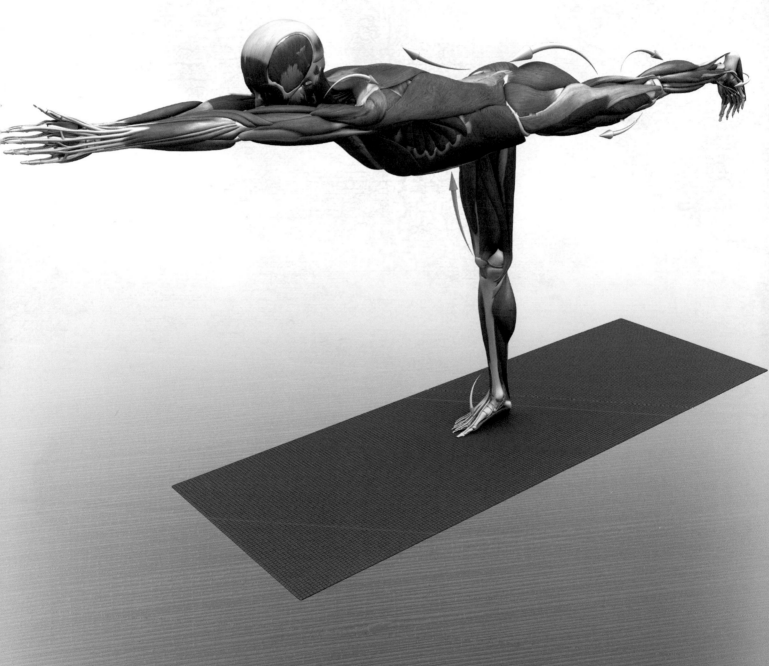

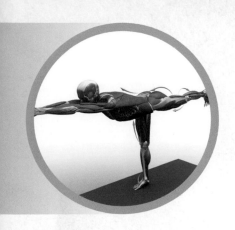

Virabhadrasana III Preparation

Begin by using a wall or chair for support and balance. Bend the standing leg and keep the pelvis aligned over the ankle. Raise the torso directly up by contracting the quadriceps to straighten the knee, like a hydraulic lift. Firmly engage the raised-leg buttocks and lower back muscles as well as the quadriceps to straighten the knee and lift the leg. Bend the standing leg to lower the center of gravity if you lose your balance. Gradually work toward practicing the pose away from the wall.

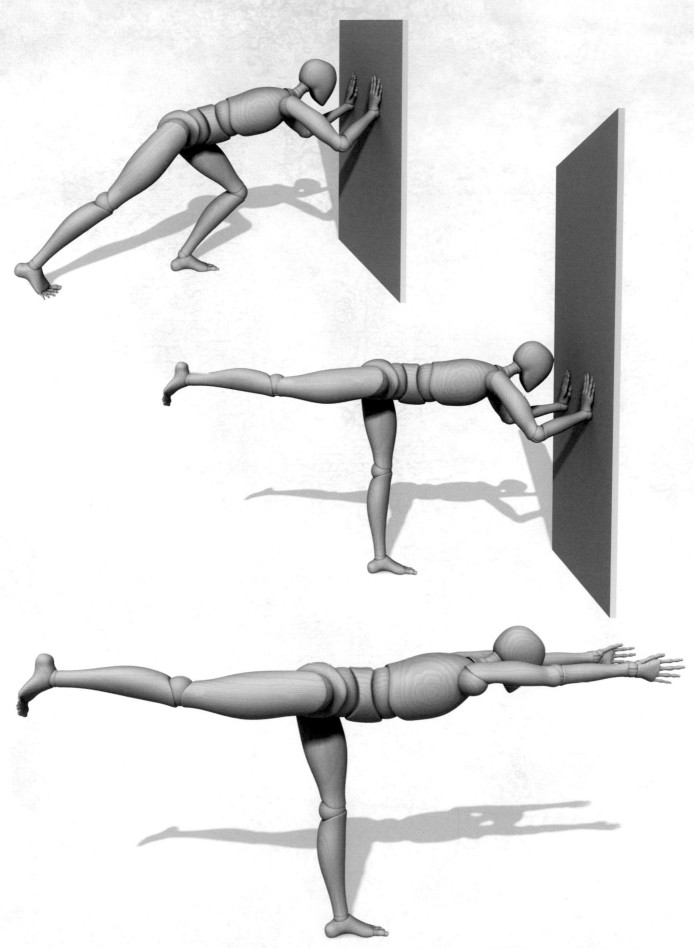

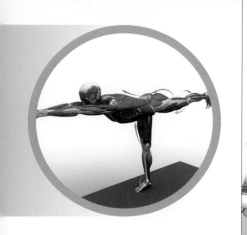

STEP 1 Flex the torso over the standing leg by engaging the psoas and pectineus. Remember that the sartorius and rectus femoris muscles cross the hip and can be used to synergize the main hip flexors. You will activate the rectus femoris when you contract the quadriceps to straighten the knee. If the kneecap rolls inward, externally rotate the thigh to contract the sartorius muscle.

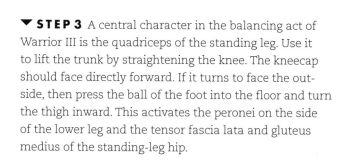

STEP 2 Look at the interconnections among the back, hip, and knee extensors in this pose. The quadriceps, synergized by the tensor fascia lata, extend the raised knee. The gluteus maximus, synergized by the adductor magnus, extends the raised hip and tilts the pelvis backwards. Engage the gluteus maximus and adductor magnus by contracting the buttocks and drawing the back foot toward the midline. Activating the gluteus maximus also externally rotates the leg, an undesirable effect in the final pose. Counter this by engaging the tensor fascia lata and gluteus medius muscles to internally rotate the hip. A cue for this is to visualize pressing the outside of the raised foot against an imaginary wall to create an abduction force and access the secondary action of internal rotation. This returns the leg to neutral, with the kneecap facing down. Arch the back to engage the erector spinae and quadratus lumborum muscles and lift the trunk.

▼ **STEP 3** A central character in the balancing act of Warrior III is the quadriceps of the standing leg. Use it to lift the trunk by straightening the knee. The kneecap should face directly forward. If it turns to face the outside, then press the ball of the foot into the floor and turn the thigh inward. This activates the peronei on the side of the lower leg and the tensor fascia lata and gluteus medius of the standing-leg hip.

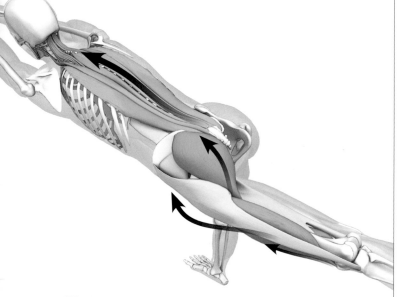

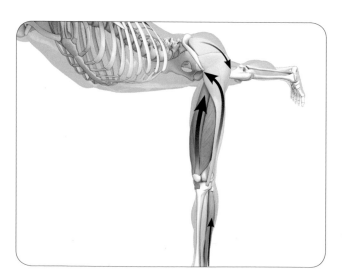

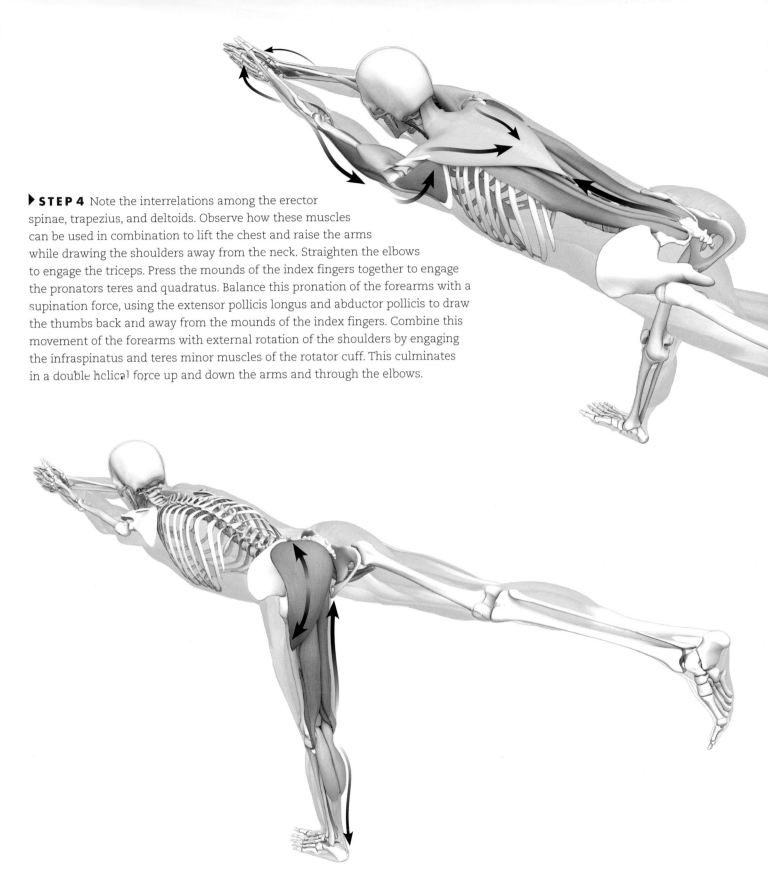

▶ STEP 4 Note the interrelations among the erector spinae, trapezius, and deltoids. Observe how these muscles can be used in combination to lift the chest and raise the arms while drawing the shoulders away from the neck. Straighten the elbows to engage the triceps. Press the mounds of the index fingers together to engage the pronators teres and quadratus. Balance this pronation of the forearms with a supination force, using the extensor pollicis longus and abductor pollicis to draw the thumbs back and away from the mounds of the index fingers. Combine this movement of the forearms with external rotation of the shoulders by engaging the infraspinatus and teres minor muscles of the rotator cuff. This culminates in a double helical force up and down the arms and through the elbows.

▲ SUMMARY All of these actions combine to create an intense stretch in the muscles at the back of the standing leg and hip—the gastrocnemius/soleus complex, the hamstrings, and the gluteus maximus. Remember that activating the antagonist muscle groups (the quadriceps and psoas and their synergists) creates reciprocal inhibition of the muscles that are lengthening in this pose, protecting them and allowing them to relax into the stretch.

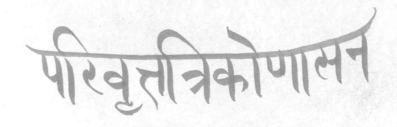

PARIVRTTA TRIKONASANA

REVOLVING TRIANGLE POSE

IN PARIVRTTA TRIKONASANA THE SHOULDERS ROTATE IN ONE DIRECTION AND the pelvis in another. We connect these opposing rotational actions to create movement in the spine. At the same time, the lower side of the body contracts and the upper side of the body expands. Eccentrically contract the muscles of the upper side of the torso to prevent the ribcage from bulging. Stabilize the core of the pelvis and expand the chest forward toward the front leg. Balancing rotation and expansion in this way turns the body into a storehouse for potential energy.

BASIC JOINT POSITIONS

- The back foot turns in 30 degrees and supinates.
- The front foot turns out 90 degrees.
- The back hip extends.
- The front hip flexes.
- Both knees extend.
- The trunk laterally flexes and rotates.

- The upper shoulder externally rotates and abducts.
- The lower shoulder internally rotates and abducts.
- The cervical spine rotates to turn the head to face upward.

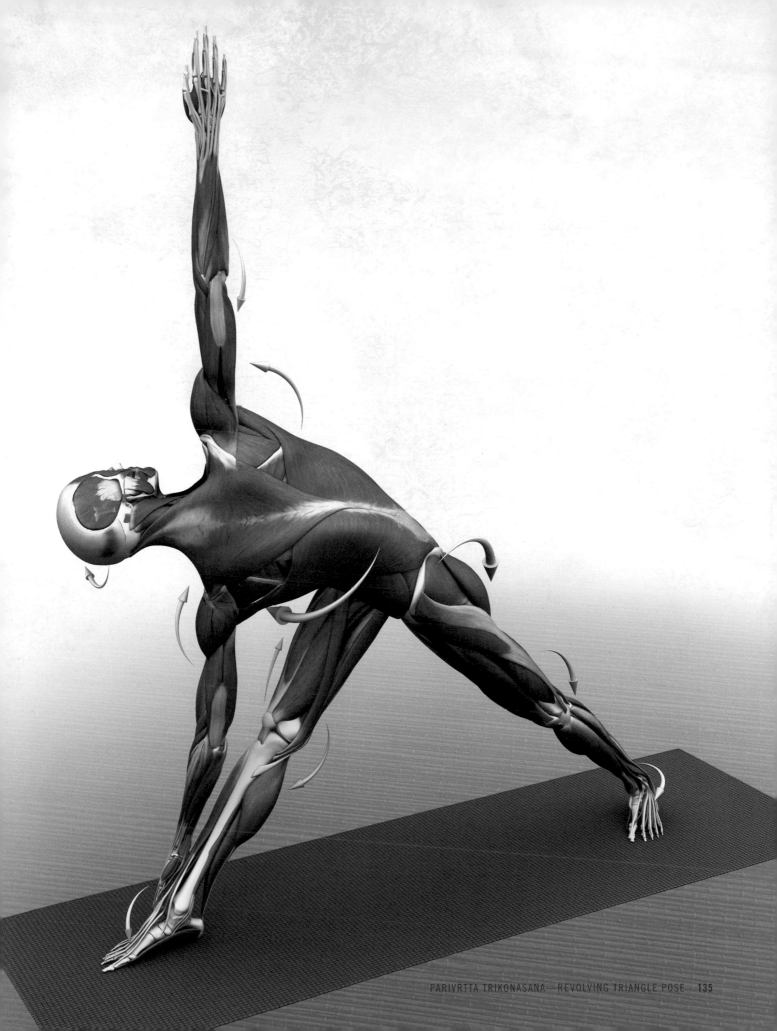

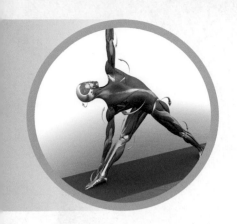

Parivrtta Trikonasana Preparation

Start by bending the forward knee. Reach down with the opposite-side hand and grasp the lower leg. Fixing the hand in place, bend the elbow to turn the body toward the leg. Do this by contracting the biceps. Then slide the hand down the outside of the leg while at the same time straightening the knee. Use a block in the beginning. Press down on the block with the lower-side arm and note how this turns the chest. Raise the upper arm and draw the upper-side shoulder blade toward the spine to create more rotation in the upper side of the chest. Eventually place the hand on the outside of the ankle or onto the floor, and use the entire arm to revolve the body.

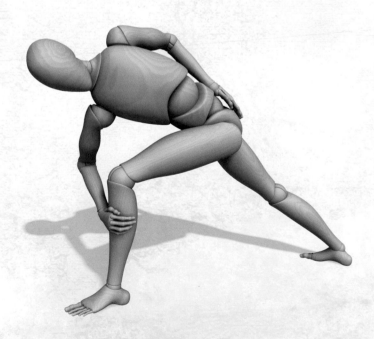

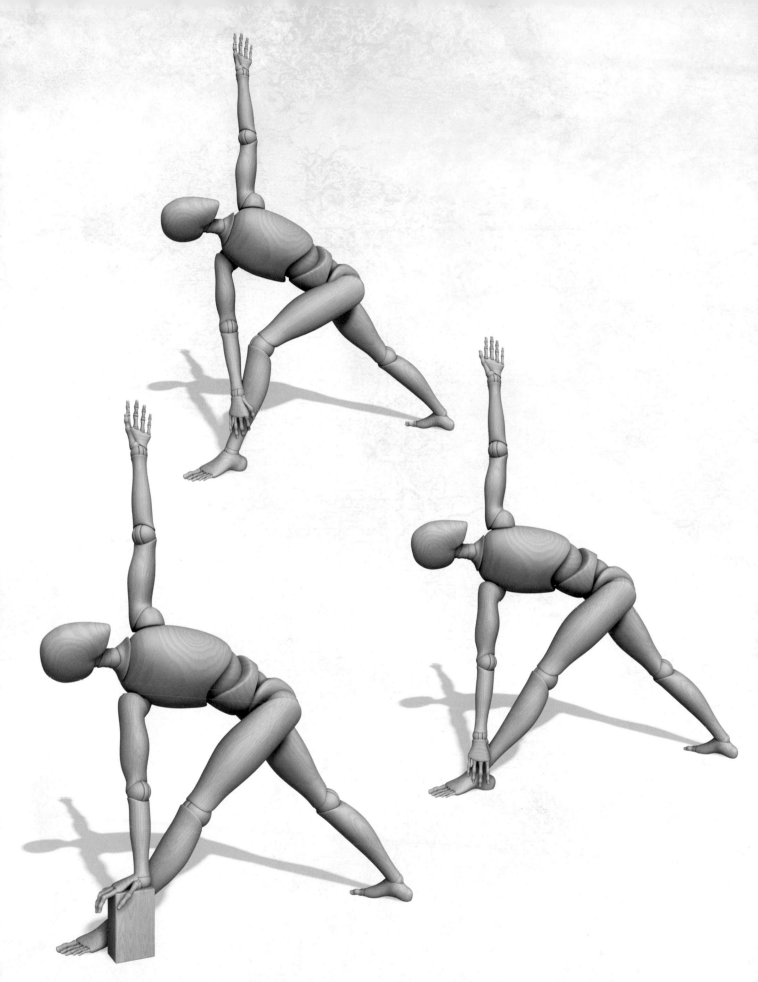

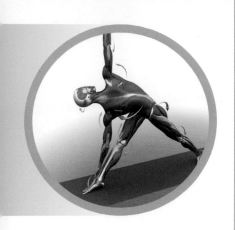

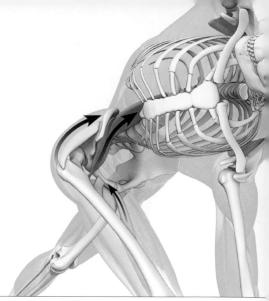

STEP 1 Squeeze the trunk against the front thigh to contract the hip flexors. This activates the psoas muscle differently than in the previous poses because the pelvis is rotated further. Visualize the front-leg gluteus minimus. This muscle refines flexion of the hip when the femur and pelvis are oriented in this fashion.

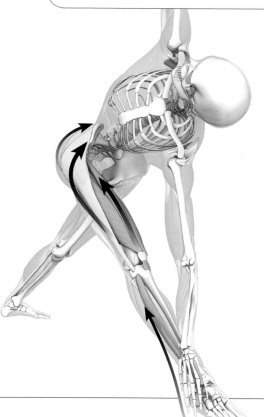

◀STEP 2 Activate the quadriceps to straighten the knee. Press the front foot into the floor, balancing your body weight across the sole. Typically the weight shifts to the outer edge of the foot in this pose. Activate the peronei to counter this by creating an eversion force at the ankle, and distribute the weight back onto the ball of the foot. Contract the hip abductors by attempting to drag the front foot toward the lower-side hand. Note how this closed chain contraction of the tensor fascia lata and gluteus medius shifts the pelvis to align it with the leg.

STEP 3 Use the lower-side external oblique and upper-side internal oblique muscles of the abdomen to turn the trunk. Activate the upper-side erector spinae to arch the back slightly. Press down into the floor with the arm, abducting the scapula and activating the serratus anterior muscle. A cue that I use for this is to imagine pushing the hand against a wall. Connect these actions to the upper arm by contracting the triceps to extend the elbow. Note how these muscles combine to turn the body deeper into the pose.

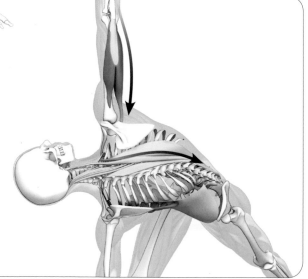

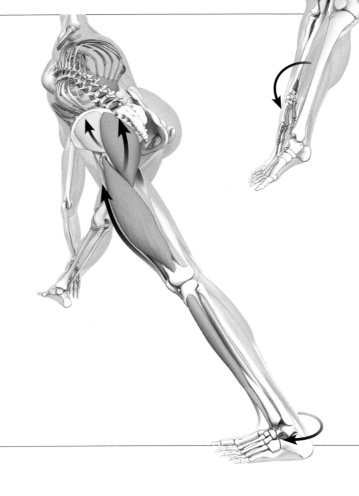

▶ **STEP 4** Press the palm of the lower-side hand against the outside of the ankle, pronating the forearm. This engages the pronators teres and quadratus. Use the triceps to extend the elbow. Contract the posterior third of the deltoid to further extend the arm and press the hand against the ankle. This turns the body from the core of the shoulder girdle. Connect these actions to the upper-side arm by contracting the rhomboids to draw the scapula toward the midline.

STEP 5 Engage the quadriceps to straighten the back knee and press the heel into the floor. Use the remainder of the foot to refine your balance. Activate the tibialis anterior and posterior muscles of the lower leg to turn the foot inward and dorsiflex the ankle (draw the top of the foot toward the shin). Counter this internal rotation of the foot by engaging the gluteus maximus and medius to extend and externally rotate the hip. This creates a coiled double helix through the leg, connecting the floor with the pelvis. Note how engaging the gluteus maximus turns the pelvis in an opposite direction to the shoulders. The actions of the shoulders turning in one direction and the pelvis in another combine to rotate the spine.

◀ **SUMMARY** This pose focuses a stretch on the front-leg hamstrings and gluteus maximus, but other muscles are also being stretched, including the back-leg hamstrings and gastrocnemius/soleus, the upper-side abdominal obliques, and to a lesser extent, the pectoralis major. Straightening the arms stretches the biceps and brachialis muscles.

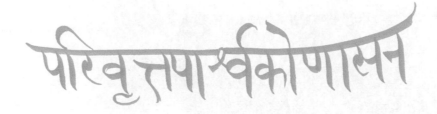

PARIVRTTA PARSVAKONASANA

REVOLVING LATERAL ANGLE POSE

PARIVRTTA PARSVAKONASANA IS BOTH A TWIST AND A STANDING POSE. TWO STORIES take place simultaneously here: lunging forward and turning the torso. The main story in this pose is the combined action of turning the shoulders in one direction and the pelvis in the other; the connection between the shoulders and the pelvis turns the spine. Press the upper arm into the thigh to create a leveraging force that rotates the torso toward the front leg. At the same time, externally rotate the rear hip and leg to turn the lower body in the other direction. This produces a coiling effect on the vertebral column. As with the warrior poses, Parivrtta Parsvakonasana has the front hip and knee flexing to produce a sense of forward movement, while the back hip and knee extend to constrain this momentum. Combine the leveraging forces of the extremities with the rotational force produced by the abdominal oblique muscles to turn the torso and spine.

The skeletal system is divided into the axial and appendicular skeletons, with the appendicular skeleton being further divided into the arms and shoulder girdle (upper section) and the legs and pelvic girdle (lower section). The axial skeleton comprises the vertebral column and thorax. Just as the earth revolves around its axis, when you connect the upper and lower appendicular skeletons, as in this pose, you can rotate the body around its axis—the vertebral column (see *The Key Muscles of Yoga* for a more detailed explanation on the skeletal system).

BASIC JOINT POSITIONS

- The back foot rotates inward 90 degrees.
- The front foot turns out 90 degrees.
- The front hip and knee flex to 90 degrees.
- The back hip extends and externally rotates.
- The trunk laterally flexes and rotates.
- The wrists extend and the elbows flex.
- The shoulders abduct.
- The cervical spine rotates to turn the head to face upward.

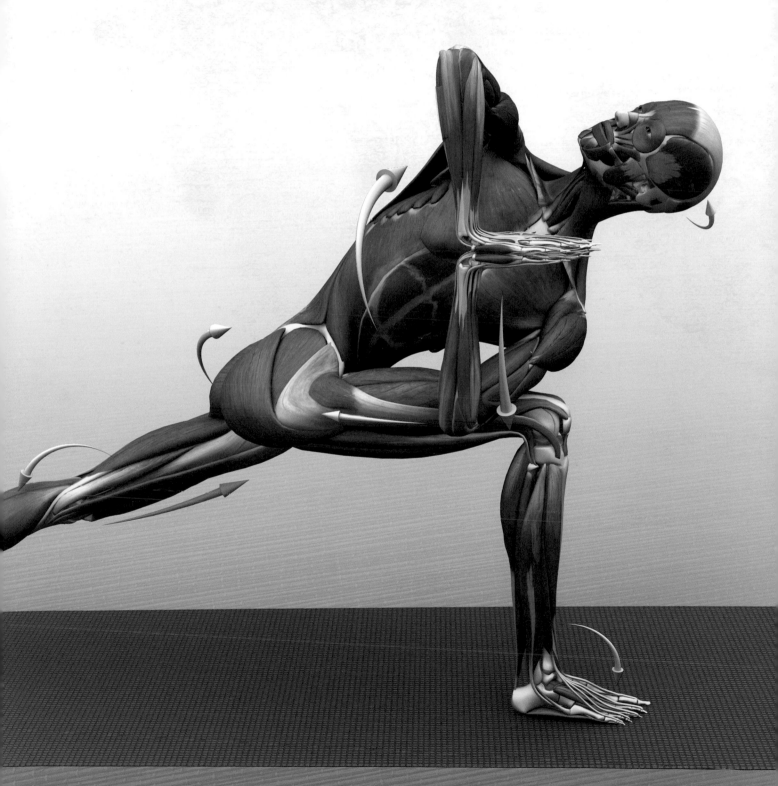

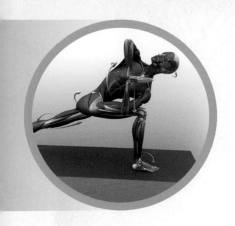

Parivrtta Parsvakonasana Preparation

Begin in a lunge position with the back knee on the floor. Keeping the knee on the floor provides an opportunity to feel the lunge and twisting actions in the pose without the challenge of balance. Press the opposite elbow against the front knee to turn the torso. Activate the abdominals to get a feeling for rotating the trunk toward the front leg. Contract the back-leg quadriceps and gluteus maximus to straighten the knee and extend the hip.

As flexibility increases with time, place the forward hand on a block and press the back of the arm against the outer thigh. The classical pose has the hand on the floor outside of the foot and the back foot flat on the floor, turning in about thirty degrees. This requires a great deal of flexibility in the spine and should never be forced.

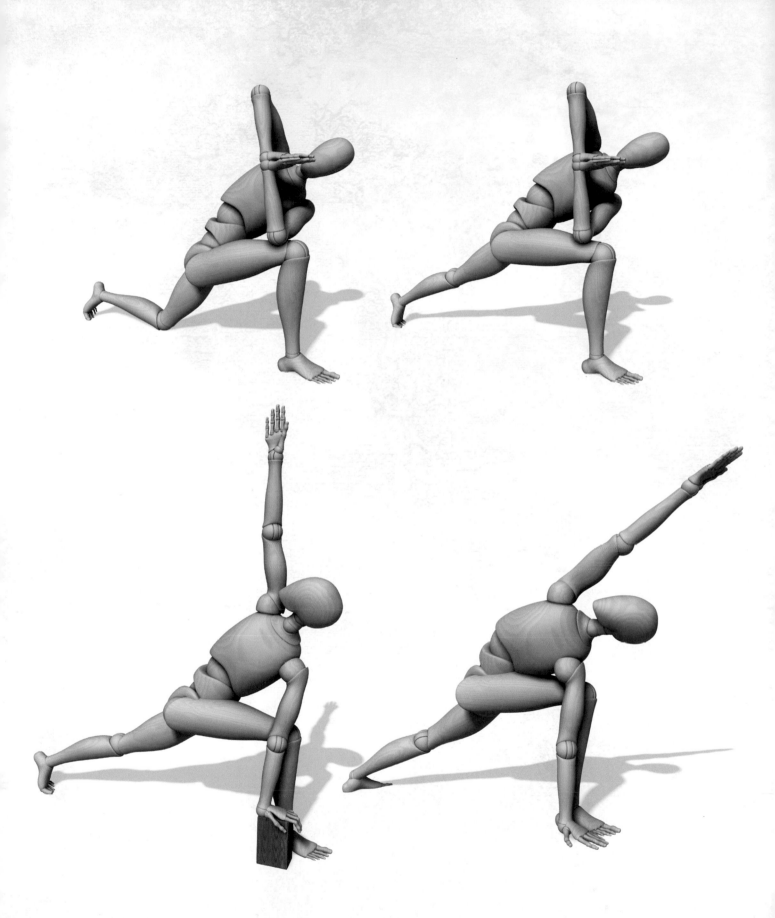

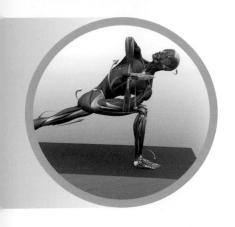

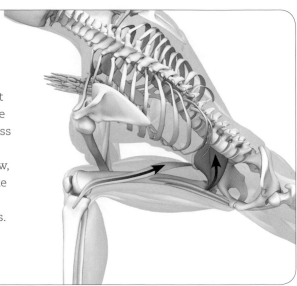

STEP 1 Squeeze the torso against the thigh to contract the hip flexors, including the psoas and its synergists. Press the outer side of the thigh against the back of the elbow, activating the sartorius. Note that the pelvis tilts forward as the front-leg femur flexes.

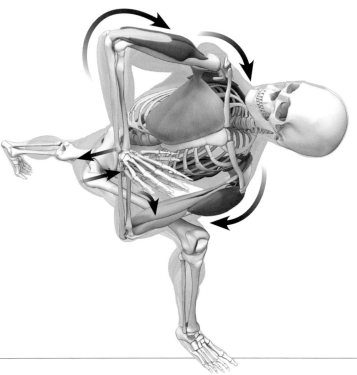

◀ **STEP 2** Press the elbow against the knee to turn the body. Break down this act into the following subplots, and feel how each action deepens the twist of the torso:

A. Press the upper palm down against the lower palm to activate the upper-side pectoralis major.

B. Press the back of the lower arm into the thigh to activate the lower-side posterior deltoid.

C. With the front arm fixed against the thigh, draw the upper-side scapula toward the spine. The rhomboids will pull the torso into a deeper rotation around the axis of the spine.

D. Attempt to scrub the upper-side palm away from the body to contract the triceps and the lower-side palm toward the chest to contract the biceps. The palms won't move because they are pressing together, but the activation of these muscles aids to turn the torso.

STEP 3 Engage the lower-side abdominal oblique muscles to revolve the trunk toward the front leg. At the same time, gently arch the back to turn the torso from the core. The lower-side serratus anterior muscles aid to rotate the torso, and the upper-side rhomboids draw the scapula toward the spine to synergize this action. These combined movements turn the chest around the axis of the spine.

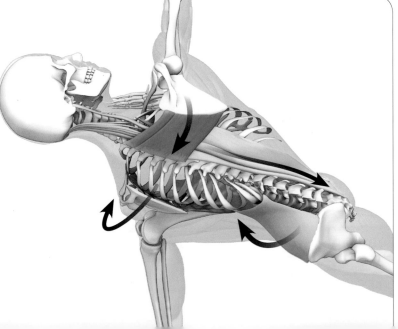

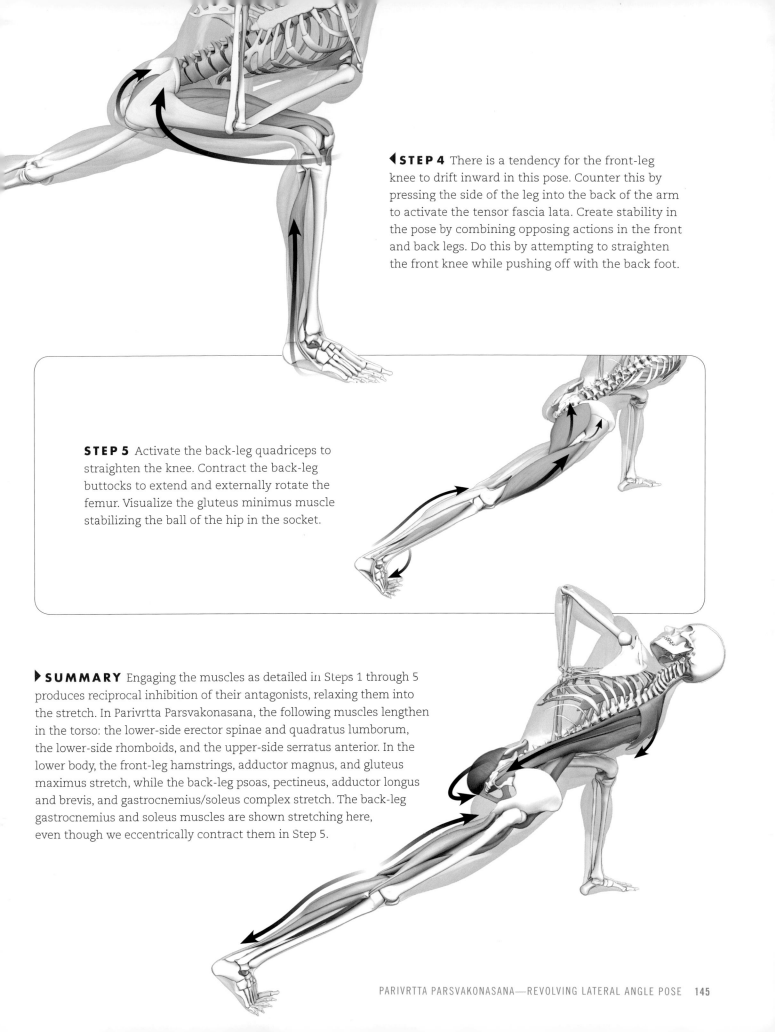

◀ STEP 4 There is a tendency for the front-leg knee to drift inward in this pose. Counter this by pressing the side of the leg into the back of the arm to activate the tensor fascia lata. Create stability in the pose by combining opposing actions in the front and back legs. Do this by attempting to straighten the front knee while pushing off with the back foot.

STEP 5 Activate the back-leg quadriceps to straighten the knee. Contract the back-leg buttocks to extend and externally rotate the femur. Visualize the gluteus minimus muscle stabilizing the ball of the hip in the socket.

▶ SUMMARY Engaging the muscles as detailed in Steps 1 through 5 produces reciprocal inhibition of their antagonists, relaxing them into the stretch. In Parivrtta Parsvakonasana, the following muscles lengthen in the torso: the lower-side erector spinae and quadratus lumborum, the lower-side rhomboids, and the upper-side serratus anterior. In the lower body, the front-leg hamstrings, adductor magnus, and gluteus maximus stretch, while the back-leg psoas, pectineus, adductor longus and brevis, and gastrocnemius/soleus complex stretch. The back-leg gastrocnemius and soleus muscles are shown stretching here, even though we eccentrically contract them in Step 5.

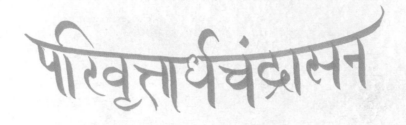

PARIVRTTA ARDHA CHANDRASANA

REVOLVING HALF-MOON POSE

PARIVRTTA ARDHA CHANDRASANA MERGES BALANCING WITH TWISTING. AS with Parivrtta Trikonasana and Parivrtta Parsvakonasana, the shoulder girdle and pelvis move in opposite directions, connected by the revolving spinal column. Initially we use the hand on the floor for stability; as balance in the pose improves, press the hand into the mat and use it to lever the body deeper into the twist. Work to align the femur over the tibia and ankle, so that the bone strength supports the weight of the body while perpendicular to the floor. Raise and lower the pelvis to work with the center of gravity and maintain balance. If you waver or start to fall, bend the standing-leg knee and/or lower the raised leg from the hip to regain stability. Extend the upper arm straight up into the air and use it to lever the upper-side chest into the twist. Create a line of action extending back through the raised-leg heel to constrain the body back, and then open the chest forward in the opposite direction. This creates an energetic coil from the heel to the top of the head. Pelvic stability is the key to success in this pose. Obtain this by engaging the psoas of the standing leg and the gluteus maximus of the raised leg. These two opposing actions create a helical force across the pelvis, tethering it in place and minimizing wavering in the pose.

BASIC JOINT POSITIONS

- The standing hip flexes.
- The trunk laterally flexes and rotates.
- The back hip extends.
- Both knees extend.
- Both shoulders abduct and externally rotate.
- The cervical spine rotates to turn the head to face upward or forward.

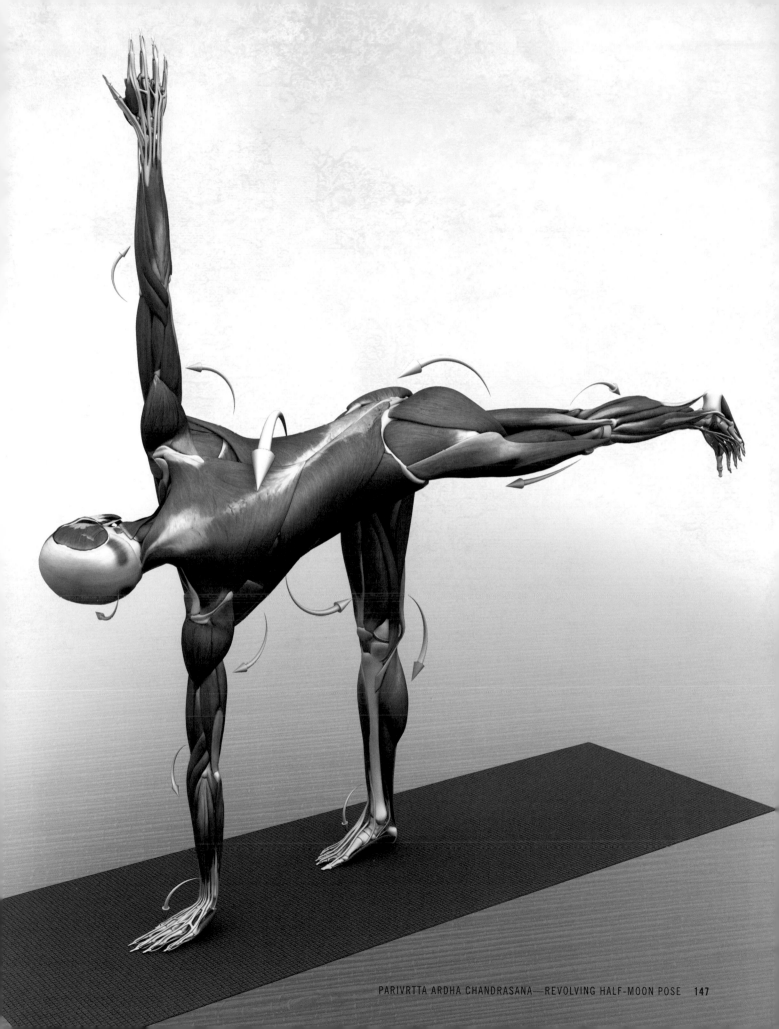

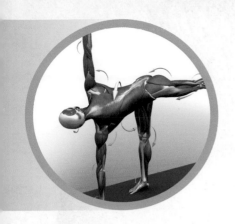

Parivrtta Ardha Chandrasana Preparation

Bend the front knee and grasp the outside of the lower leg with the hand, as with Parivrtta Trikonasana. Bend the elbow to lever the torso into a twist against the thigh. Roll the upper shoulder back and raise the upper arm to turn the chest.

Next, walk the back foot toward the front, and at the same time, bring the lower-side hand a few inches ahead of the front foot. Pause for a moment in this position. Maintain the torso turning and squeezing against the front thigh; this engages the hip flexors, including the psoas. With the standing leg bent, tilt the torso down while contracting the gluteal muscles to raise the back leg like a teeter totter. Squeeze the buttocks muscles to lift the leg parallel to the floor. Simultaneously contracting these two muscles—the psoas and the gluteus maximus—stabilizes the pelvis. Finally, activate the quadriceps to straighten the knee and lift the torso like the action of a hydraulic lift.

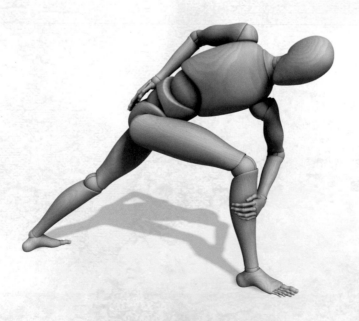

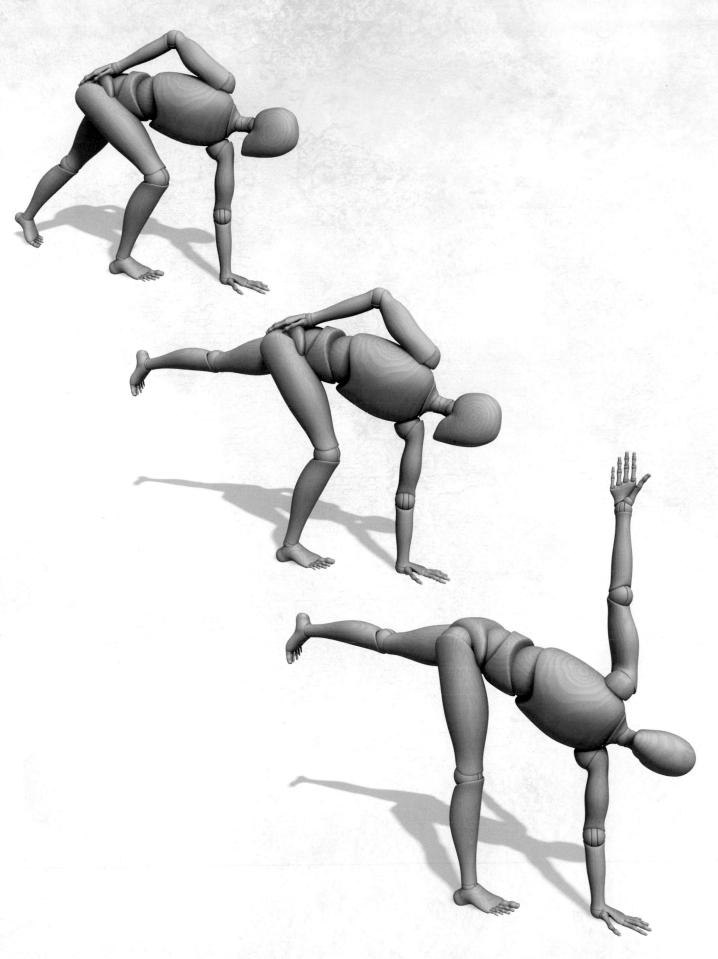

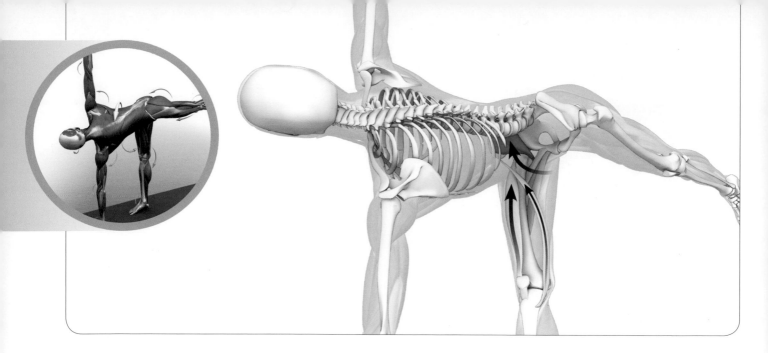

▲ **STEP 1** Engage the hip flexors, including the psoas, pectineus, and adductors longus and brevis, to bend the torso over the standing leg. Bend from the pelvis rather than rounding the back to come into the pose. Engage the quadriceps to straighten the standing leg. Contracting this muscle group automatically activates the rectus femoris, a subpart of the quadriceps. The rectus femoris and sartorius cross the pelvis and knee and synergize the psoas to flex the trunk over the leg. These polyarticular muscles all cross multiple joints; this creates a connection that extends from the lumbar spine to the lower leg.

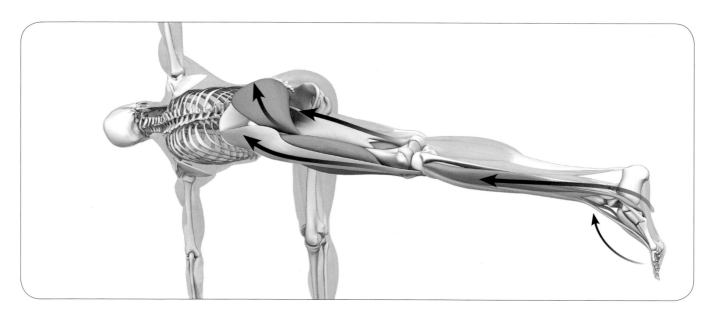

▲ **STEP 2** Lift the back leg by contracting the gluteus maximus, the prime mover of hip extension. This muscle also externally rotates the femur. In this pose, we want the kneecap to face directly down. To accomplish this we need to counteract the external rotation caused by the gluteus maximus contracting. Do this by activating the tensor fascia lata and gluteus medius to internally rotate the femur. A cue for this is to imagine pressing the outer edge of the back foot against a wall. This invokes both the abduction and internal rotation components of the tensor fascia lata and gluteus medius and illustrates "dual action" of a muscle. When you try this cue, don't let your leg abduct to the side. Instead, engage the adductor magnus to resist this action. The adductor magnus also synergizes the gluteus maximus in extending the hip. Straighten the knee by engaging the quadriceps. The already contracted tensor fascia lata helps to straighten the knee. The peroneus longus and brevis on the side of the lower leg engage to evert and open the sole of the foot backwards.

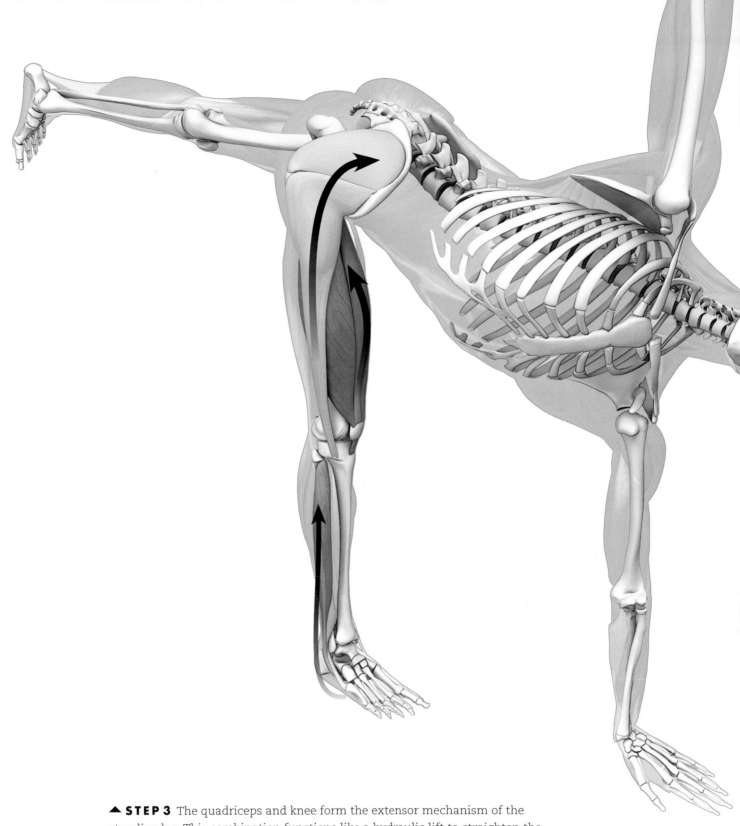

▲ **STEP 3** The quadriceps and knee form the extensor mechanism of the standing leg. This combination functions like a hydraulic lift to straighten the knee and lift the pelvis in this pose. When we stand on one leg, the gluteus medius automatically contracts to tether the pelvis in place. The tensor fascia lata along the side of the leg synergizes both this action and that of straightening the knee. Align the femur over the tibia and ankle, so that the weight is supported by the arch of the foot. Activate the arch by contracting the peronei at the side of the lower leg to press the ball of the foot into the floor.

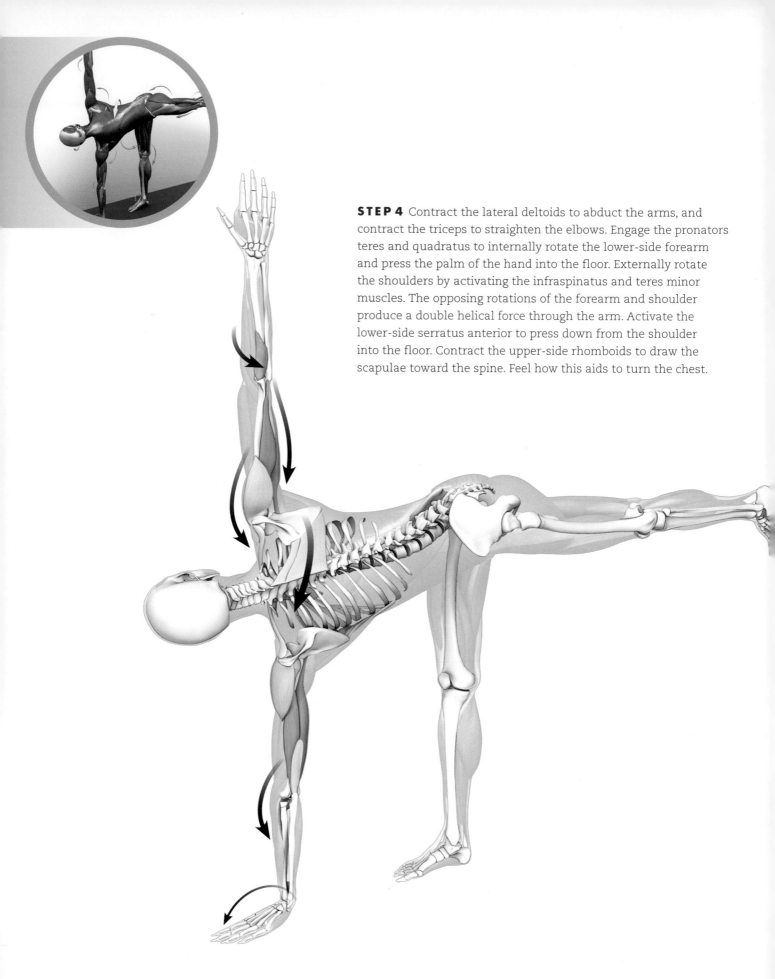

STEP 4 Contract the lateral deltoids to abduct the arms, and contract the triceps to straighten the elbows. Engage the pronators teres and quadratus to internally rotate the lower-side forearm and press the palm of the hand into the floor. Externally rotate the shoulders by activating the infraspinatus and teres minor muscles. The opposing rotations of the forearm and shoulder produce a double helical force through the arm. Activate the lower-side serratus anterior to press down from the shoulder into the floor. Contract the upper-side rhomboids to draw the scapulae toward the spine. Feel how this aids to turn the chest.

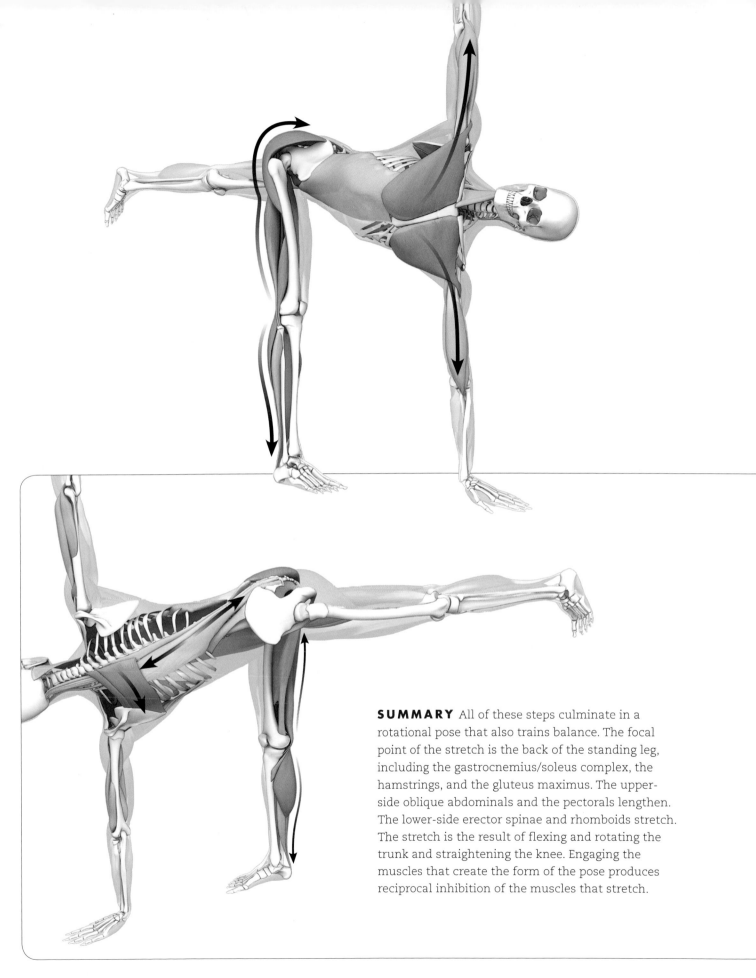

SUMMARY All of these steps culminate in a rotational pose that also trains balance. The focal point of the stretch is the back of the standing leg, including the gastrocnemius/soleus complex, the hamstrings, and the gluteus maximus. The upper-side oblique abdominals and the pectorals lengthen. The lower-side erector spinae and rhomboids stretch. The stretch is the result of flexing and rotating the trunk and straightening the knee. Engaging the muscles that create the form of the pose produces reciprocal inhibition of the muscles that stretch.

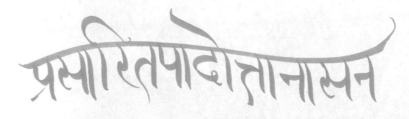

PRASARITA PADOTTANASANA

SPREAD FEET INTENSE-STRETCH POSE

SCULPTOR FREDERICK WELLINGTON RUCKSTULL SAID, "EVERYTHING IN NATURE folds at evening." Life is full of alternating opposites, such as inhaling and exhaling, sleeping versus waking, and fight or flight versus rest and digest. Each of these dualities demonstrates a dynamic balancing of opposites. Sequencing in yoga can be used to exaggerate a cycle of expansion and contraction. We begin with poses that open the front of the body and close with poses that draw the energy inward. At the conclusion of the standing series, we fold forward into Prasarita Padottanasana to relax. Note that this pose is also an inversion, in that it places the head below the heart and stimulates the pressure receptors in the heart, aorta, and carotid arteries. This shifts the autonomic nervous system from fight or flight to rest and digest.

We can use triangulation to locate the focus of the stretch, here the hamstrings and gastrocnemius/soleus complex, extending into the erector spinae and quadratus lumborum muscles of the back. Flex the trunk forward while extending the knees to create two vertices of the triangle. Flexing forward draws the ischial tuberosities (the origin of the hamstrings) upward. Extending the knees draws the insertion of the hamstrings away from their origin. This action also draws the origin of the gastrocnemius away from its insertion on the Achilles tendon. The third corner of the triangle is the stretch at the backs of the legs and the trunk.

Attempting to draw the hands forward when they are fixed on the mat brings the trunk deeper into the pose and lifts the ischial tuberosities higher; this deepens the hamstring stretch. This is an example of using a subplot, in this case flexing the elbows and shoulders, to contribute to the main story of the pose (flexing the trunk forward and straightening the knees).

Add a physiological component to these biomechanical actions by engaging the quadriceps to stimulate reciprocal inhibition of the hamstrings, causing them to relax into the stretch. Finally, balance eversion and inversion of the ankles by simultaneously contracting the peroneus longus and brevis and tibialis posterior muscles. This creates stillness and stability at the foundation of the pose.

BASIC JOINT POSITIONS

- The feet are parallel.
- The knees extend.
- The trunk flexes.
- The elbows flex.
- The shoulders flex forward, adduct, and depress.

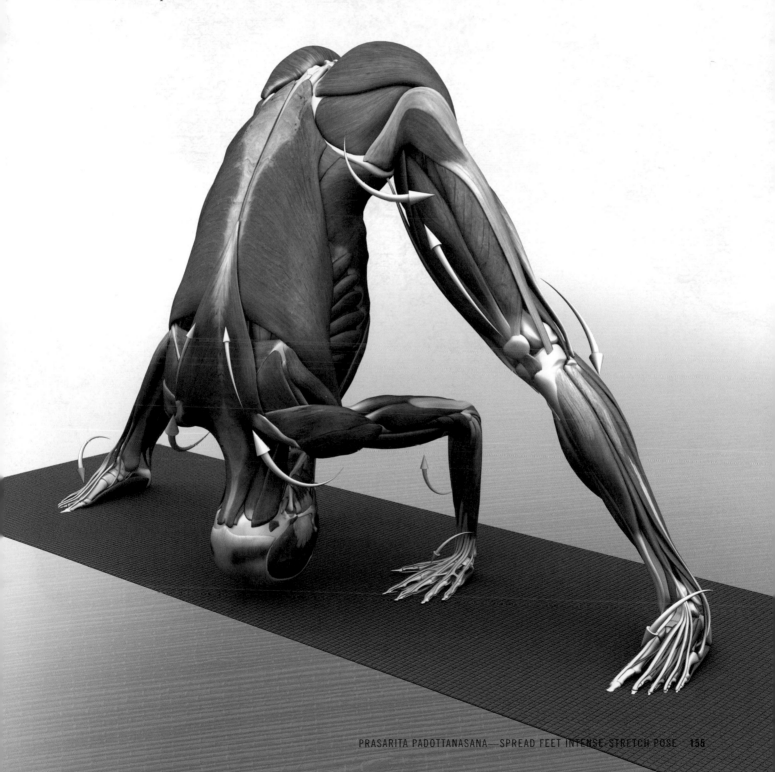

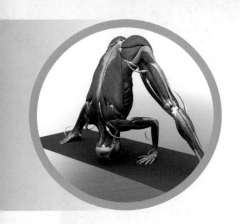

Prasarita Padottanasana
Preparation

Begin with the hands on the hips and the feet spread apart. Activate the quad-riceps to straighten the knees. You can use the cue of "lifting the kneecaps" to bring awareness to this action. Flex the knees slightly as you bend forward to release the hamstrings at their insertions on the lower legs, and note how you can draw your trunk deeply into the pose. Engage the hip flexors and abdominals to squeeze the torso against the thighs. Fix the hands on the mat and bend the elbows to draw the trunk deeper. Hold the trunk in place and engage the quadri-ceps to straighten the knees. Stabilize the ankles by pressing the balls of the feet into the mat, while at the same time lifting the arches. Bend the knees to safely come out of the pose.

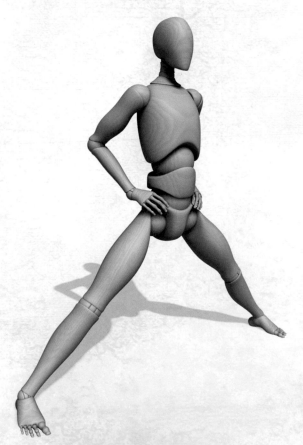

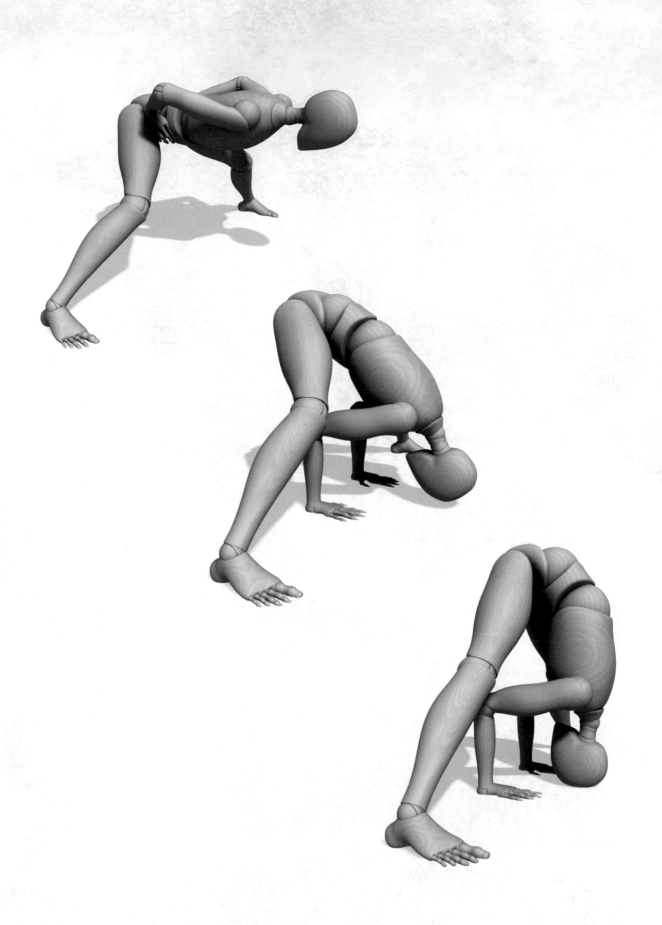

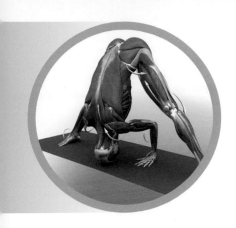

STEP 1 Engage the psoas and its synergists to flex the hips and draw the trunk forward over the legs. Then squeeze the abdominals to activate the rectus abdominis. Contracting these muscles creates reciprocal inhibition of the gluteus maximus, quadratus lumborum, and erector spinae muscles, allowing them to relax into the stretch. Note that when the femurs flex, the pelvis tilts forward, drawing the ischial tuberosities up.

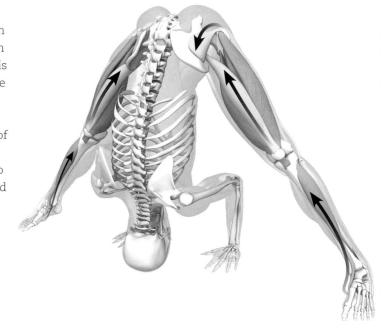

STEP 2 Activate the tibialis anterior and posterior to turn the feet in (inversion) and lift the arches. Balance inversion of the ankles with a slight eversion force. The cue for this is to press the balls of the feet into the floor. This engages the peroneus longus and brevis muscles at the outside of the lower legs to stabilize the ankles. Contract the quadriceps to straighten the knees. This creates reciprocal inhibition of the hamstring muscles at the backs of the legs. When the hips are flexing, the gluteus minimus acts as a synergist to the psoas and also internally rotates the hips, as illustrated here. Visualize this muscle creating these actions.

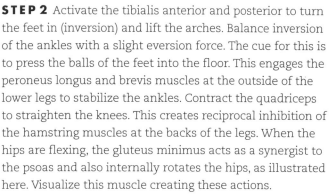

STEP 3 Press the mounds at the base of the index fingers into the floor. This calls on the pronators teres and quadratus to internally rotate the forearms. Contract the wrist flexors to press the hands into the mat. Then attempt to bend the elbows by engaging the biceps and brachialis muscles. Because the hands are fixed on the mat, the force of this contraction is transmitted to the torso, drawing it deeper into flexion. Now, consider that the toes point forward. Engage the anterior deltoids and attempt to drag the palms forward on the mat as if to raise the arms overhead. The force of this contraction draws the torso deeper into the pose. The elbows tend to drift outward here. Engage the pectoralis major to adduct the elbows, and note how this synergizes the forward flexion of the torso. All of this illustrates how a secondary action of the shoulders and arms can be used to affect the primary focus of the stretch at the backs of the legs.

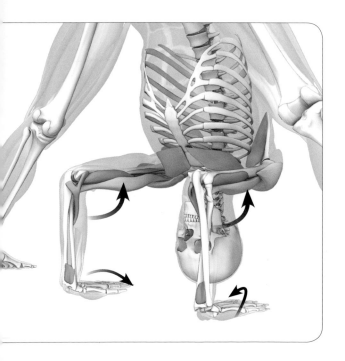

STEP 4 Press the palms into the mat and attempt to rotate them externally, like washing a window. This cue activates the infraspinatus and teres minor muscles of the rotator cuff and externally rotates the humeri. Draw the shoulders away from the ears, using the lower third of the trapezius. Note how these two actions—externally rotating the shoulders and drawing them away from the ears—open the chest forward and deepen the flexion of the trunk.

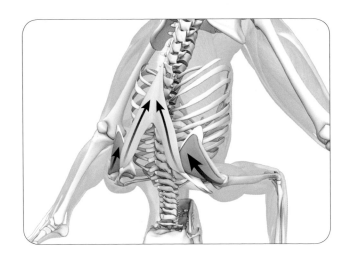

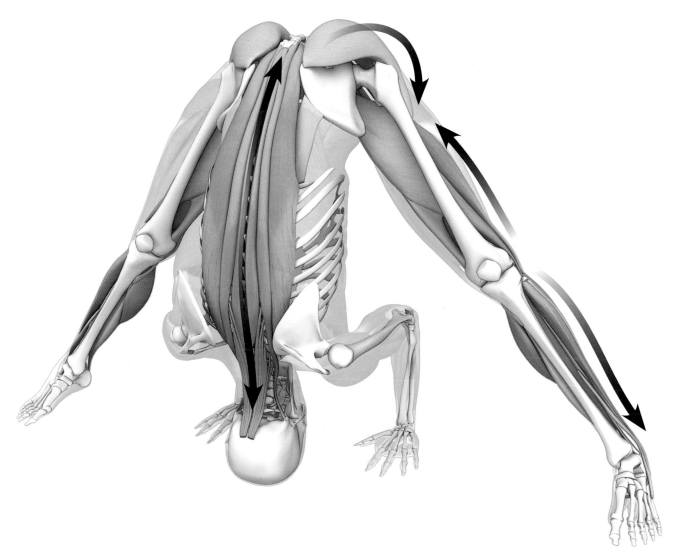

▲ **STEP 5** Combine these steps to stretch the entire posterior kinetic chain, including the gastrocnemius/soleus complex and the hamstring, adductor magnus, gluteus maximus, quadratus lumborum, and erector spinae muscles. Inverting the feet (turning them inward) stretches the muscles that evert the feet, the peroneus longus and brevis. Eccentrically contract these muscles to stabilize the ankles. Remember that the prime movers of the pose activated in Steps 1 and 2 initiate reciprocal inhibition of the muscles that stretch here.

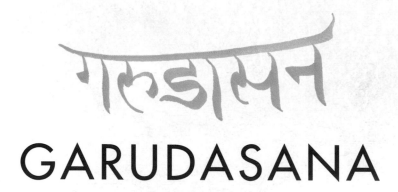

GARUDASANA

EAGLE POSE

EARLY IN THE STANDING POSE SEQUENCE WE HAD TREE POSE, WHICH OPENS THE hips outward and lifts the chest upward. At the conclusion of the series, we fold the body forward in Prasarita Padottanasana and then consolidate and draw the energy inward with Garudasana. Consider Garudasana to be a balancing version of the fetal position, with the hips adducted and internally rotated and the arms crossed over one another. Three plots take place simultaneously in Garudasana, each synergizing the other: the arms adduct across the chest; the legs adduct in front of the pelvis, with the femurs internally rotating; and the feet form the foundation for a balancing act. Squeezing the legs together connects the pelvis with the feet and helps to maintain balance. Squeezing the elbows together augments the contractile force of the leg muscles and the pelvic diaphragm, thereby synthesizing balance and mula bandha.

BASIC JOINT POSITIONS

- The standing knee flexes 20 degrees.
- Both hips adduct and internally rotate.

- The back extends.
- The shoulders flex to 90 degrees and adduct.
- The elbows flex.

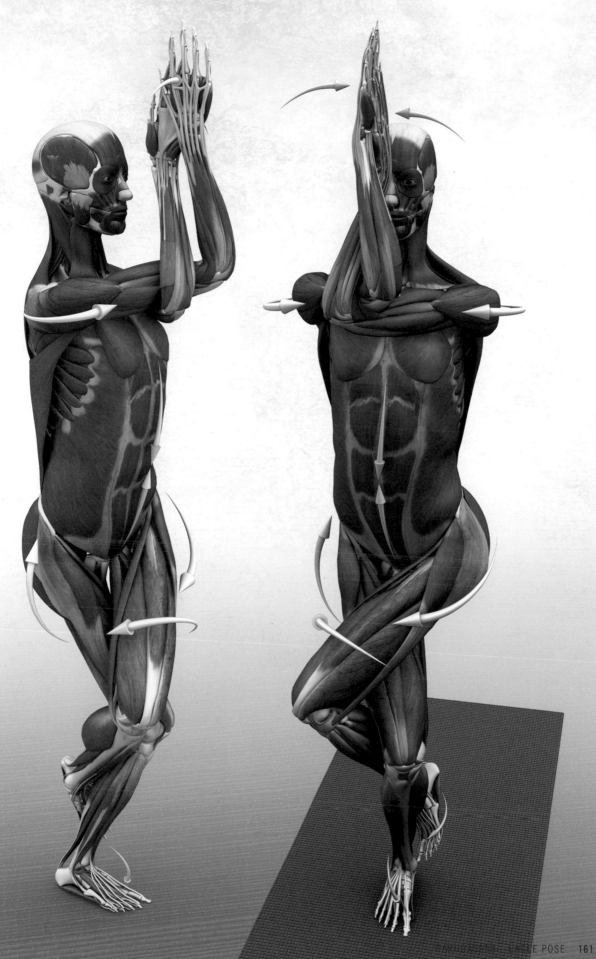

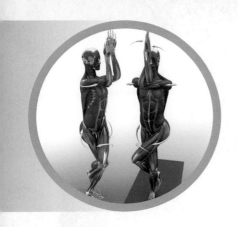

Garudasana Preparation

Begin by adducting the elbows and cross one over top of the other. Squeeze the lower elbow into the upper one. Then cross the hands and press the fingers of the lower hand into the palm of the upper hand. If you're unable to bring your hands into this position, simply cross the elbows and press them together. With time and improved flexibility, work toward bringing the hands into the crossed-over position.

Next, bend the knees. This lowers the center of gravity and strengthens the muscles of the thighs. Bring the opposite leg over the thigh. Use opposites between the upper and lower body; for example, if the left arm crosses on top of the right, then the right leg crosses on top of the left, and vice versa. Squeeze the thighs together. Finally, hook the foot around the lower leg as shown. If you lose balance, bend the knees to lower the center of gravity and regain stability. Use twisting poses like Ardha Matsyendrasana (Half Lord of the Fishes Pose) to stretch the abductor muscles of the hips.

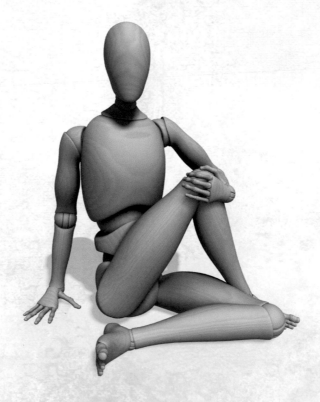

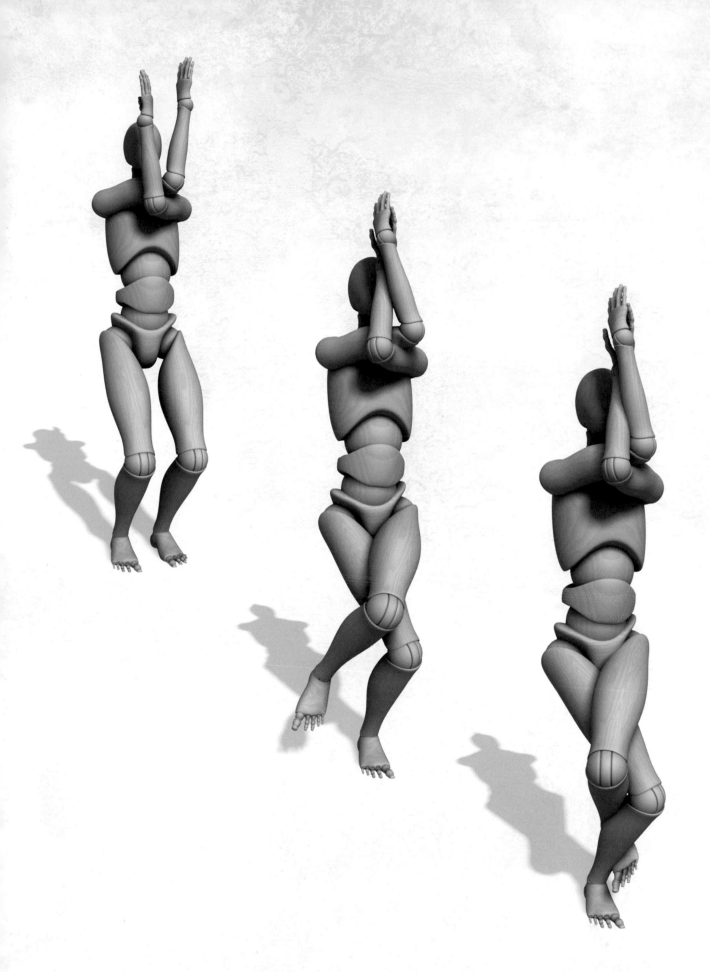

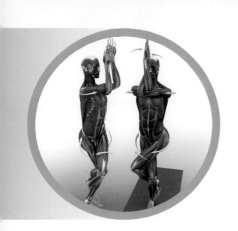

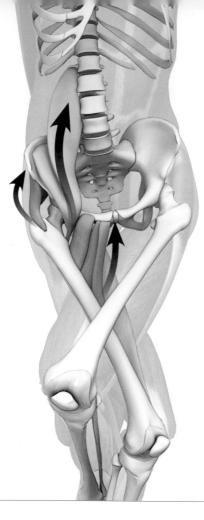

STEP 1 Flex and adduct the standing leg. The psoas major straightens the lumbar spine and combines with the iliacus muscle to flex the femur and tilt the pelvis forward. The pectineus and anterior adductors synergize each other to adduct the femur. The gluteus minimus (shown here at the side of the pelvis) flexes and internally rotates the hip and stabilizes the femur in the hip socket. Visualize these muscles in action when doing the pose.

STEP 2 Balancing on one leg involves a dynamic interplay among the muscles located from the hip to the foot. When you're standing upright, the femur and tibia are relatively aligned, so some of the body weight is taken up by the tensile strength of the bones. When the knee bends, the bones no longer align and the weight is supported by the extensor mechanism of the knee (the quadriceps, patella, and patellar tendon).

The gluteus medius and tensor fascia lata perform two actions here. First, both muscles automatically engage to tether and stabilize the pelvis. Second, they internally rotate the thigh. Contract the tensor fascia lata by pressing the outside of the knee into the top leg. This stabilizes the pose.

Finally, distribute your weight evenly across the sole of the foot. Balance inversion and eversion of the foot by engaging the tibialis posterior muscle and the peroneus longus and brevis muscles, respectively. The actions of these lower leg muscles stabilize the ankle and dynamize the arch of the foot.

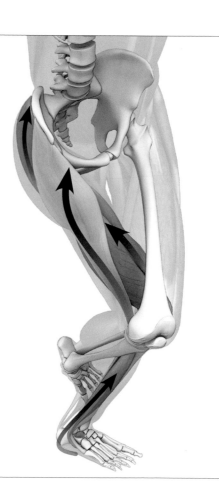

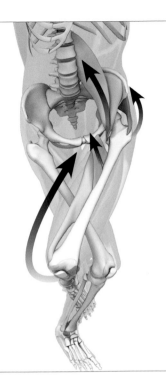

STEP 3 Draw the upper leg across the lower by engaging the psoas and the adductor group. Flex the femur and stabilize it in the hip socket by visualizing the gluteus minimus contracting. This muscle also internally rotates the flexed femur. Squeeze the thighs together by engaging the adductor muscles of both legs. Polish and dynamize the pose by attempting to draw the adducted femurs apart; this engages the tensor fascia lata, as detailed in Step 2.

▶ **STEP 4** Hook the upper foot around the lower leg and dorsiflex it by drawing the top of the foot into the calf. This activates the tibialis anterior muscle and toe extensors at the front of the leg. Evert the foot by contracting the peronei on the side of the leg. Balance this with slight inversion of the foot by engaging the tibialis posterior muscle to stabilize the ankle.

Press the ball of the foot into the floor to assist in balance. This engages the peroneus longus and brevis muscles of the standing leg. At the same time, engage the tibialis posterior of the standing leg to dynamize the arch of the foot.

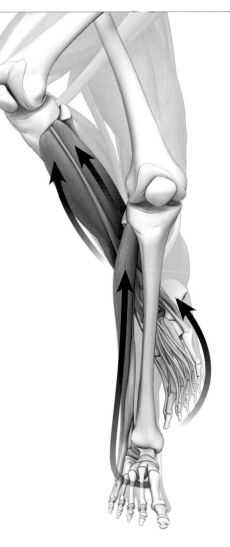

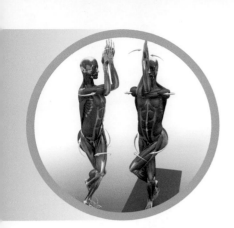

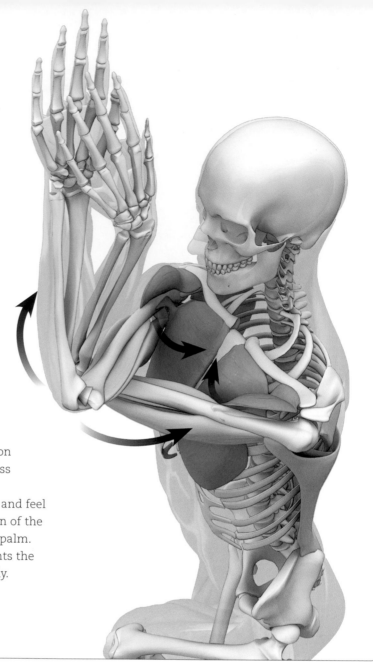

STEP 5 Contract the pectoralis major as you draw the arms toward one another, adducting the shoulders. The latissimus dorsi, teres major, and long head of the triceps assist in this action. Create an opposing force by attempting to lower the arms while engaging the anterior deltoids to resist this movement. A cue for this action is to squeeze the elbows together, bringing awareness to the latissimus dorsi at the back of the body.

Attempt to straighten the elbows while resisting and feel how this activates the triceps, refining the adduction of the arms across the chest. Squeeze the fingers into the palm. Activating these muscles in the upper body augments the force of contraction of the muscles in the lower body.

▶ **STEP 6** Adduct the arms in front of the chest to stretch the rhomboids and middle trapezius on the back. Gently arch the back by engaging the erector spinae and quadratus lumborum muscles. Draw the back of the ribcage down and expand it by engaging the serratus posterior (visualization helps in this action). Activate the standing-leg gluteals to balance the pelvis. These muscles combine with the psoas at the front of the hip to stabilize the femur in the socket.

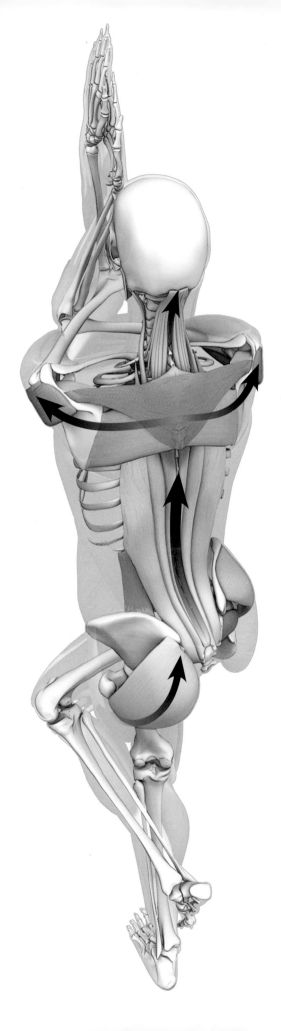

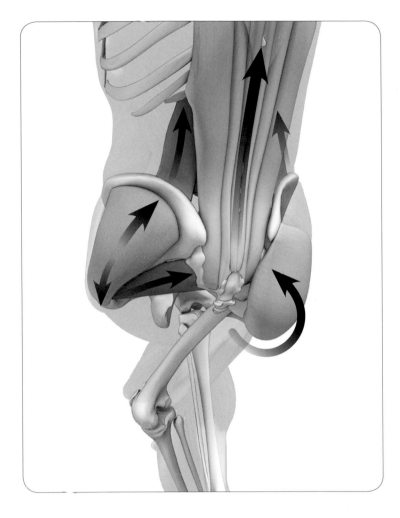

STEP 7 Notice how adducting and internally rotating the upper leg stretches the abductor component of the gluteus medius and tensor fascia lata, as well as the piriformis, obturators internus and externus, superior and inferior gemelli, and quadratus femoris muscles (the deep external rotators of the hip).

RESTORATIVE POSES
SUPPORTED SETU BANDHA BRIDGE POSE

Restorative poses can be used to relax the body and mind at the end of your practice. Use supported Setu Bandha to passively stretch the psoas and quadriceps. Note that this is also an inversion. It places the lower body above the heart, improving cardiac blood return and stimulating the parasympathetic division of the autonomic nervous system. This can aid to lower the heart rate and blood pressure.

Press down through the feet, contracting the quadriceps to lift the torso up. Place the block under the sacrum (and not under the lumbar). Rest the weight evenly on the block and keep the knees bent, as shown here. Place a folded blanket under the head to hold the neck in a slightly flexed position, and let the arms fall out to the side with the palms facing up. Close the eyes and relax here for several minutes. Then lift up off the block, place the pelvis on the floor, and roll to the right side, resting in the fetal position before getting up.

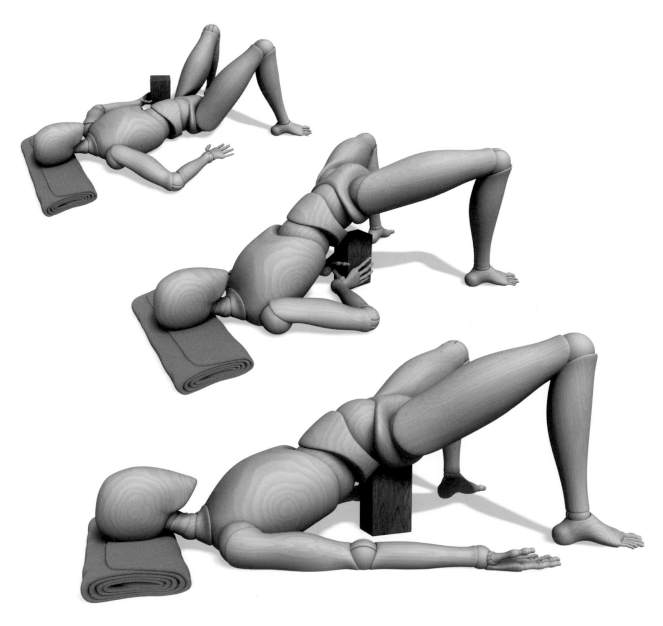

VIPARITA KARANI LEGS-UP-THE-WALL POSE

This restorative pose can be used at the end of your practice or after supported Setu Bandha. It passively stretches the hip extensors, such as the gluteus maximus, and opens the chest. Viparita Karani is also an inversion and has similar effects on the autonomic nervous system as supported Setu Bandha.

Place a bolster against the wall. You can put a block between the wall and the bolster to better position the pelvis so that the body does not slide off (see inset). Place a folded blanket under the head, lifting it slightly to gently flex the neck. Allow the arms to fall out to the side with the palms facing up. Close the eyes and stay here for several minutes. Then slide off the bolster, roll to the right, and rest in the fetal position for a few moments before getting up.

Lie down on your back with the head supported on a blanket and rest in Savasana.

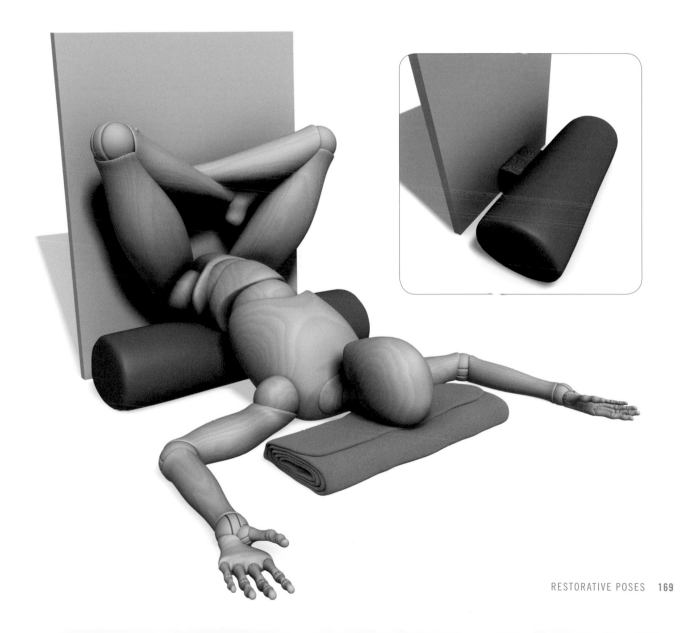

MOVEMENT
INDEX

MOVEMENT INDEX

Movements of the body have specific names. It is important to learn these names, both for teaching others yoga and for analyzing the muscles that produce the positions of the body. As a yoga teacher, it is always better to communicate your instructions in terminology that students can easily understand. Know the scientific names of the movements and have clear explanations to describe the movements in layperson's terms. Make your instructions as precise and uncomplicated as you can.

Remember that muscles contract to position the joints and appendages in the pose. If you know the joint positions, you can analyze which muscles to engage to produce the asana. With this knowledge comes the ability to use precise cues to communicate how to sculpt and stabilize the body in the pose, stretch the correct muscles, and create bandhas. Thus, unlocking the asana begins with a clear understanding of body movements.

There are six basic movements of the body: Flexion, Extension, Adduction, Abduction, Internal Rotation, and External Rotation. These movements take place in three planes, as shown here. The anatomic position is the reference point to define the direction of movement.

CORONAL PLANE: divides the body into front and back. Movements along this plane are called adduction and abduction. Adduction moves the extremity towards the midline and abduction moves the extremity away from the midline.

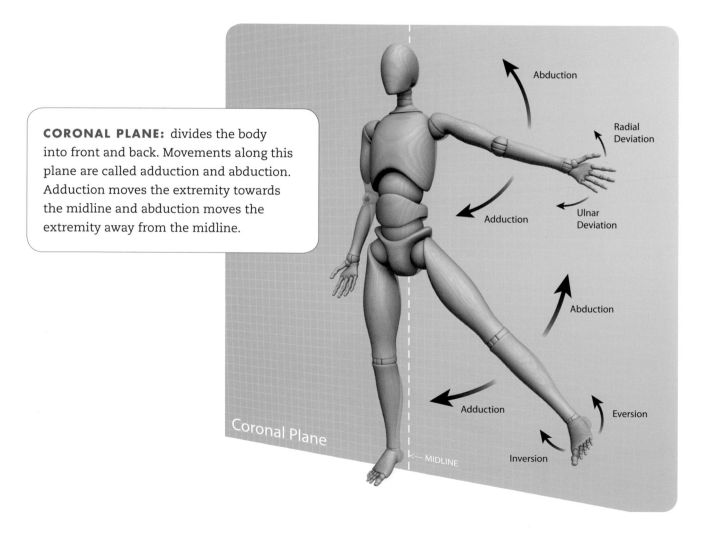

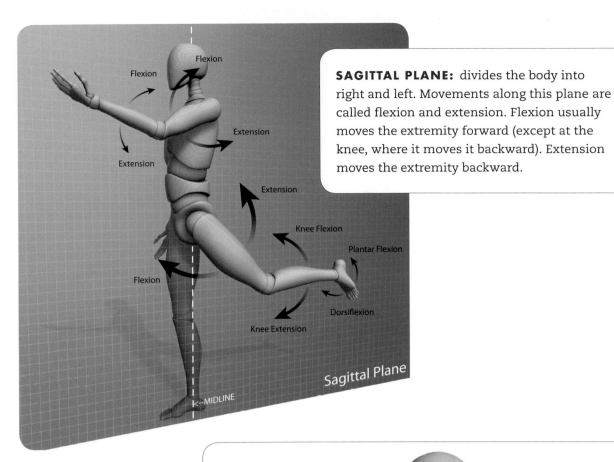

SAGITTAL PLANE: divides the body into right and left. Movements along this plane are called flexion and extension. Flexion usually moves the extremity forward (except at the knee, where it moves it backward). Extension moves the extremity backward.

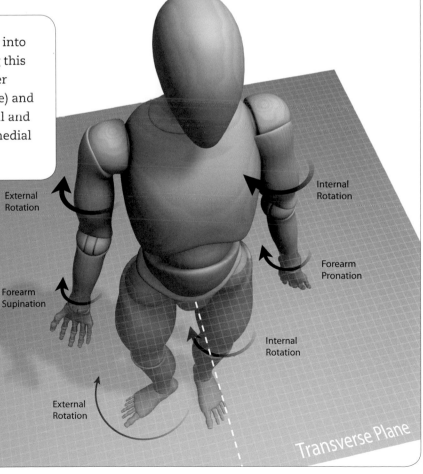

TRANSVERSE PLANE: divides the body into upper and lower halves. Movement along this plane is called rotation. Rotation is further classified as internal (towards the midline) and external (away from the midline). Internal and external rotation are also referred to as medial and lateral rotation, respectively.

MOVEMENT INDEX

Parivrtta Ardha Chandrasana and Utthita Parsvakonasana are presented as examples of how to analyze the basic joint positions in a yoga pose. The order represents the sequence of movements that create the form of the pose.

1. The standing-leg hip flexes.
2. The raised hip extends.
3. The raised knee extends.
4. The standing-leg knee extends.
5. The shoulder abducts.
6. The elbow extends.
7. The wrist extends.
8. The shoulder abducts and externally rotates.
9. The elbow extends.
10. The trunk laterally flexes and rotates.

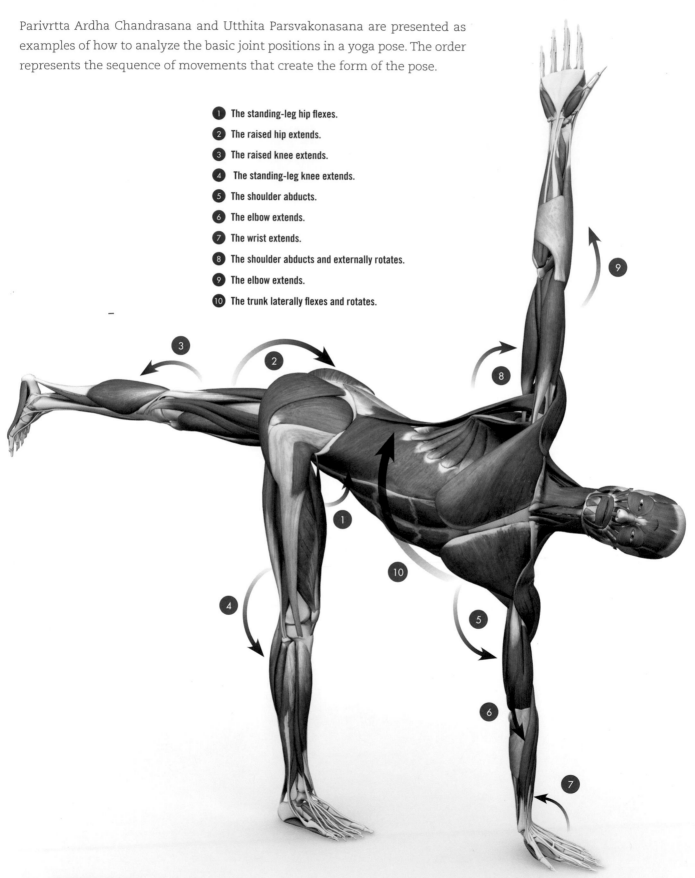

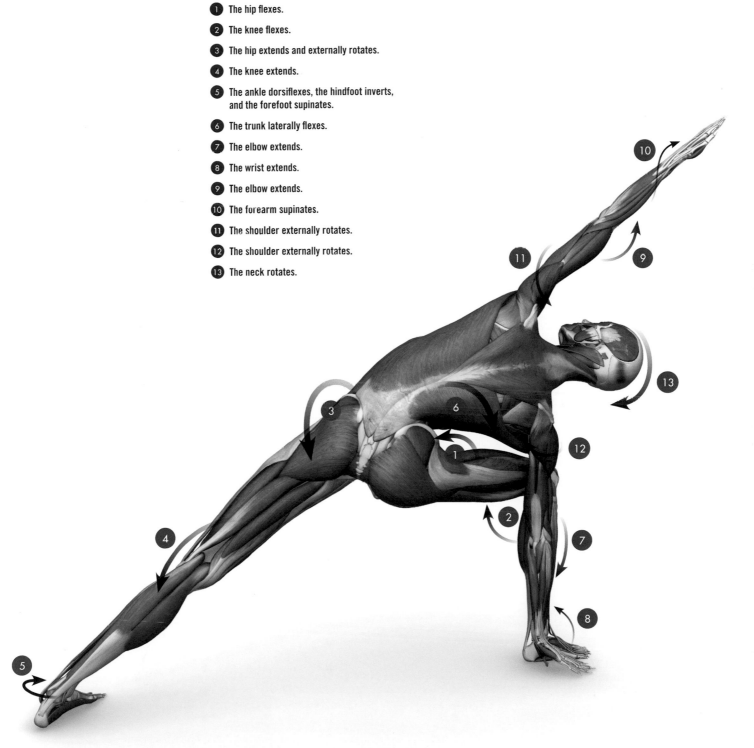

1 The hip flexes.

2 The knee flexes.

3 The hip extends and externally rotates.

4 The knee extends.

5 The ankle dorsiflexes, the hindfoot inverts, and the forefoot supinates.

6 The trunk laterally flexes.

7 The elbow extends.

8 The wrist extends.

9 The elbow extends.

10 The forearm supinates.

11 The shoulder externally rotates.

12 The shoulder externally rotates.

13 The neck rotates.

MOVEMENT TABLES

Neck

Muscle	Flexion	Extension	Lateral Flexion	Lateral Extension	Rotation
Semispinalis capitis		●	●	●	●
Splenius capitis		●	●	●	●
Sternocleidomastoid	●		●	●	●
Levator scapulae		●	●	●	
Trapezius		●	●	●	●

Trunk

Muscle	Flexion	Extension	Lateral Flexion	Rotation
External oblique	●		●	●
Internal oblique	●		●	●
Rectus abdominis	●			
Spinalis thoracis		●		
Lateral intertransversi			●	
Interspinales		●		
Longissimus thoracis		●		
Iliocostalis lumborum		●		
Multifidus		●		
Rotatores		●		●
Quadratus lumborum		●	●	
Psoas major	●		●	
Iliacus	●		●	

Hip

Muscle	Flexion	Extension	Adduction	Abduction	Internal Rotation	External Rotation
Gluteus maximus		●				●
Gluteus medius	●	●		●	●	●
Gluteus minimus	●	●		●	●	●
Tensor fascia lata	●			●	●	
Psoas major	●					●
Iliacus	●					●
Rectus femoris	●			●		
Sartorius	●			●		●
Pectineus	●		●			●
Adductor magnus		●	●			●
Adductor longus	●		●			●
Adductor brevis	●		●			●
Gracilis	●		●			●
Piriformis				●		●
Gemellus superior				●		●
Gemellus inferior				●		●
Obturator internus				●		●
Obturator externus						●
Quadratus femoris			●			●
Semitendinosus		●			●	
Semimembranosus		●			●	
Biceps femoris		●				●

MOVEMENT TABLES

Knee

Muscle	Flexion	Extension	Internal Rotation	External Rotation
Vastus medialis		●		
Vastus lateralis		●		
Vastus intermedius		●		
Rectus femoris		●		
Sartorius	●			●
Semitendinosus	●		●	
Semimembranosus	●		●	
Biceps femoris	●			●
Gracilis	●		●	
Popliteus	●			
Gastrocnemius	●			

Lower Leg

Muscle	Ankle Plantar Flexion	Ankle Dorsiflexion	Foot Eversion	Foot Inversion	Toe Flexion	Toe Extension
Gastrocnemius	●					
Soleus	●					
Tibialis anterior		●		●		
Tibialis posterior	●			●		
Peroneus longus	●		●			
Peroneus brevis	●		●			
Peroneus tertius	●		●			
Flexor digitorum longus	●			●	●	
Flexor hallucis longus	●			●	●	
Extensor digitorum longus		●	●			●
Extensor hallucis longus		●		●		●

Foot

Muscle	Toe Flexion	Toe Extension	Toe Adduction	Toe Abduction
Flexor digitorum brevis	●			
Flexor hallucis brevis	●			
Flexor digiti minimi brevis	●			
Extensor digitorum brevis		●		
Extensor hallucis brevis		●		
Abductor digiti minimi				●
Abductor hallucis				●
Adductor hallucis			●	
Lumbricales	●	●	●	
Plantar interosseus	●		●	
Dorsal interosseus	●			●

Hand

Muscle	Flexion	Extension	Adduction	Abduction
Flexor digitorum superficialis	●			
Flexor digitorum profundus	●			
Flexor pollicis longus	●			
Flexor pollicis brevis	●			
Flexor digiti minimi brevis	●			
Extensor digitorum		●		
Extensor pollicis longus		●		
Extensor pollicis brevis		●		
Extensor indicis		●		
Extensor digiti minimi		●		
Abductor pollicis longus				●
Abductor pollicis brevis				●
Adductor pollicis			●	
Abductor digiti minimi				●
Lumbricales	●	●		
Dorsal interosseus	●	●	●	

MOVEMENT TABLES

Arm and Wrist

Muscle	Elbow Flexion	Elbow Extension	Forearm Pronation	Forearm Supination	Wrist Flexion	Wrist Extension	Wrist Ulnar Deviation	Wrist Radial Deviation
Biceps brachii	●			●				
Brachialis	●							
Triceps brachii		●						
Anconeus		●						
Brachioradialis	●							
Supinator				●				
Pronator teres			●					
Pronator quadratus			●					
Extensor carpi radialis longus						●		●
Extensor carpi radialis brevis						●		●
Extensor carpi ulnaris						●	●	
Flexor carpi radialis					●			●
Flexor carpi ulnaris					●		●	
Extensor digitorum						●		
Extensor pollicis brevis								●
Extensor pollicis longus				●				●
Abductor pollicis longus								●

Shoulder

Muscle	Retraction	Protraction	Elevation	Depression	Flexion	Extension	Adduction	Abduction	Internal Rotation	External Rotation
Rhomboids	●									
Serratus anterior		●	●					●		
Trapezius	●		●	●			●	●		
Levator scapulae		●	●							
Latissimus dorsi	●			●		●	●		●	
Teres major						●	●		●	
Pectoralis major				●	●		●		●	
Pectoralis minor		●		●						
Anterior deltoid					●				●	
Lateral deltoid								●		
Posterior deltoid						●				●
Supraspinatus								●		
Infraspinatus										●
Teres minor							●			●
Subscapularis									●	
Biceps brachii					●					
Coracobrachialis					●		●			
Triceps brachii						●	●			

ANATOMY INDEX

ANATOMY INDEX
BONES

1. skull
2. mandible
3. cervical spine
4. thoracic spine
5. lumbar spine
6. sacrum
7. ilium bone (pelvis)
8. ischial tuberosity (sit bone)
9. femur
10. patella
11. tibia
12. fibula
13. ribs
14. sternum
15. clavicle
16. scapula
17. humerus
18. radius
19. ulna
20. hindfoot
21. midfoot
22. forefoot
23. carpals (wrist)
24. metacarpals
25. phalanges

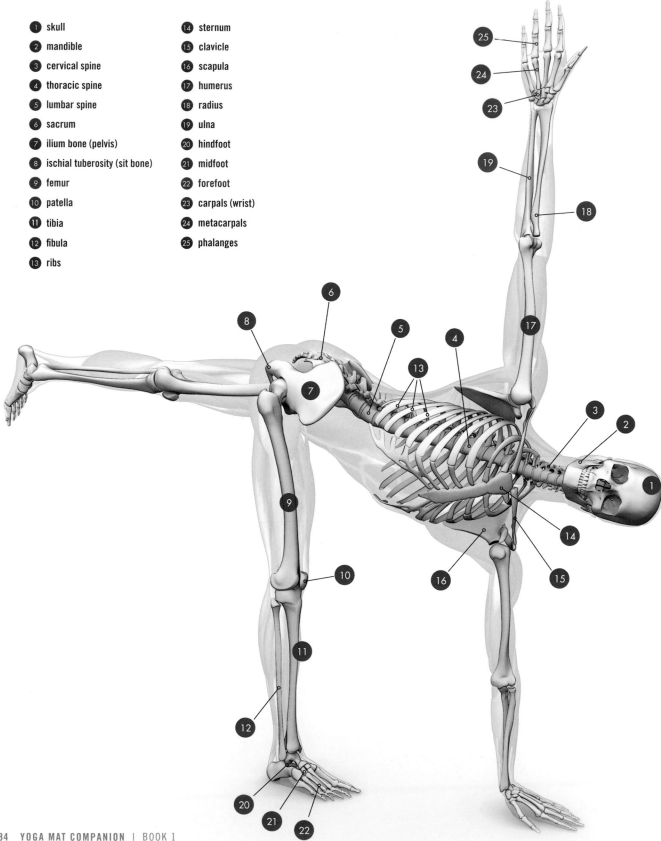

AXIAL AND APPENDICULAR SKELETONS

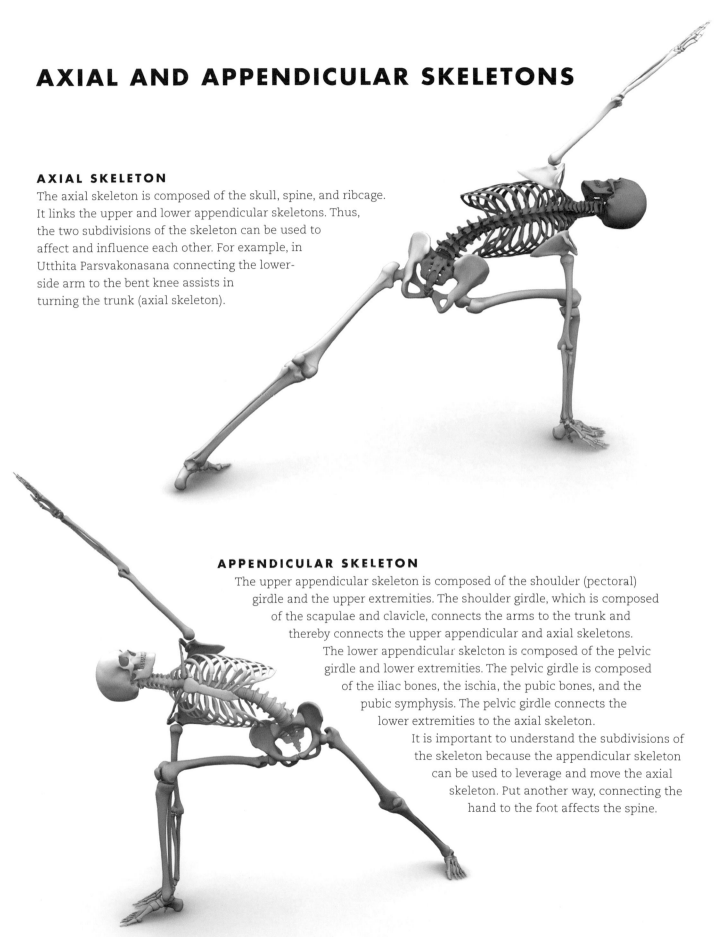

AXIAL SKELETON

The axial skeleton is composed of the skull, spine, and ribcage. It links the upper and lower appendicular skeletons. Thus, the two subdivisions of the skeleton can be used to affect and influence each other. For example, in Utthita Parsvakonasana connecting the lower-side arm to the bent knee assists in turning the trunk (axial skeleton).

APPENDICULAR SKELETON

The upper appendicular skeleton is composed of the shoulder (pectoral) girdle and the upper extremities. The shoulder girdle, which is composed of the scapulae and clavicle, connects the arms to the trunk and thereby connects the upper appendicular and axial skeletons. The lower appendicular skeleton is composed of the pelvic girdle and lower extremities. The pelvic girdle is composed of the iliac bones, the ischia, the pubic bones, and the pubic symphysis. The pelvic girdle connects the lower extremities to the axial skeleton.

It is important to understand the subdivisions of the skeleton because the appendicular skeleton can be used to leverage and move the axial skeleton. Put another way, connecting the hand to the foot affects the spine.

ANATOMY INDEX
MUSCLES

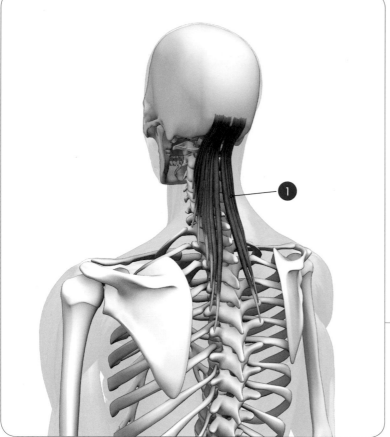

Legend

O = Origin. The proximal site where a muscle attaches to a bone.

I = Insertion. The distal site where a muscle attaches to a bone.

A = Action. The joint movement produced when the muscle contracts.

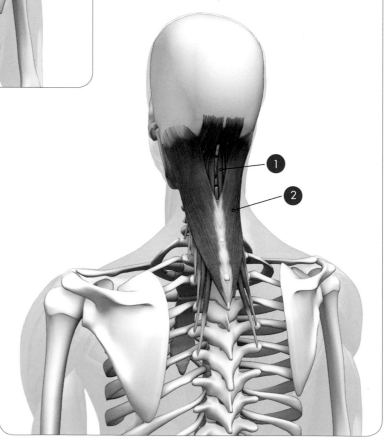

❶ Semispinalis capitis
- O: Transverse processes of lower cervical and upper thoracic vertebrae.
- I: Occipital bone.
- A: Extends head (tilts it back), assists in turning head.

❷ Splenius capitis
- O: Spinous processes of C7 and T1-4.
- I: Mastoid process of skull, behind ear.
- A: Extends head and neck; when one side contracts, laterally flexes neck; turns head toward side of individual muscle.

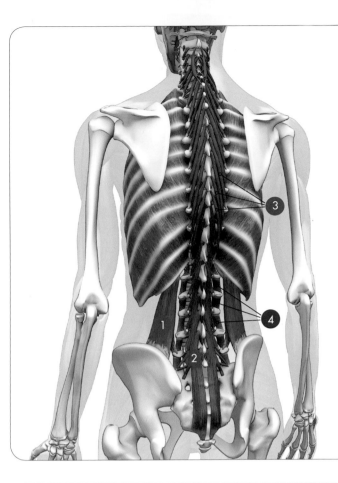

1 Quadratus lumborum

O: Posterior (back) of iliac crest.

I: Back part of rib 12, transverse processes of L1-4.

A: Laterally flexes spine (bends to side); extends and stabilizes lumbar spine; stabilizes rib 12, drawing it down during deep inhalation.

2 Multifidus

O: Back of sacrum and posterior superior iliac spine, transverse processes of lumbar, thoracic, and cervical vertebrae (all the way up the spine).

I: Two vertebrae above the vertebrae of origin; fibers are directed diagonally toward the midline and onto the spinous processes of the vertebrae of insertion.

A: Stabilizes spine during extension, flexion, and rotation.

3 Semispinalis thoracis

O: Transverse processes of T6-10.

I: Spinous processes of lower cervical and upper thoracic vertebrae.

A: Extends and rotates upper thoracic and lower cervical spine.

4 Lateral intertransversi

O: Transverse processes of lumbar vertebrae.

I: Transverse process of vertebrae immediately above vertebrae of origin.

A: Laterally flexes lumbar spine.

1 Serratus posterior superior

O: Ligamentum nuchae and spinous processes of C7-T4.

I: Ribs 2-5 on upper border.

A: Expands back of chest during deep inhalation by lifting ribs (is an accessory muscle of breathing).

2 Serratus posterior inferior

O: Spinous processes of T11-12, L1-3, thoracolumbar fascia.

I: Lower borders of ribs 9-12.

A: Stabilizes lower ribs during inhalation.

3 Spinalis thoracis

O: Transverse processes of T6-10.

I: Spinous processes of C6-7, T1-4.

A: Extends upper thoracic and lower cervical spine.

4 Longissimus thoracis

O: Posterior sacrum, spinous processes of T11-12, L1-5.

I: Transverse processes of T1-12, medial part of ribs 4-12.

A: Laterally flexes and extends spine, aids to expand chest during inhalation.

5 Iliocostalis lumborum

O: Posterior sacrum.

I: Posterior part of ribs 7-12.

A: Laterally flexes and extends lumbar spine.

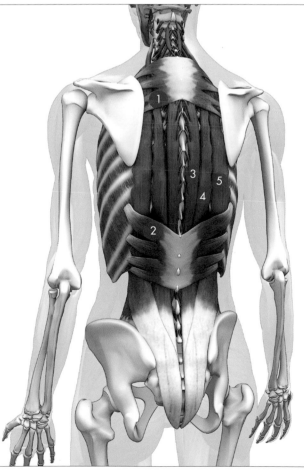

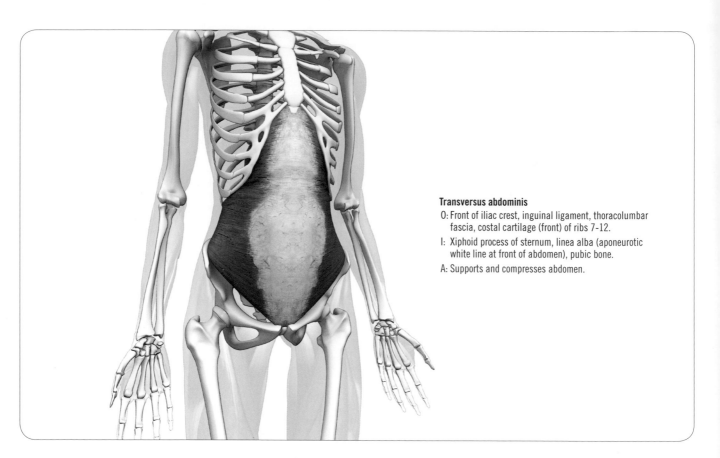

Transversus abdominis

O: Front of iliac crest, inguinal ligament, thoracolumbar fascia, costal cartilage (front) of ribs 7-12.

I: Xiphoid process of sternum, linea alba (aponeurotic white line at front of abdomen), pubic bone.

A: Supports and compresses abdomen.

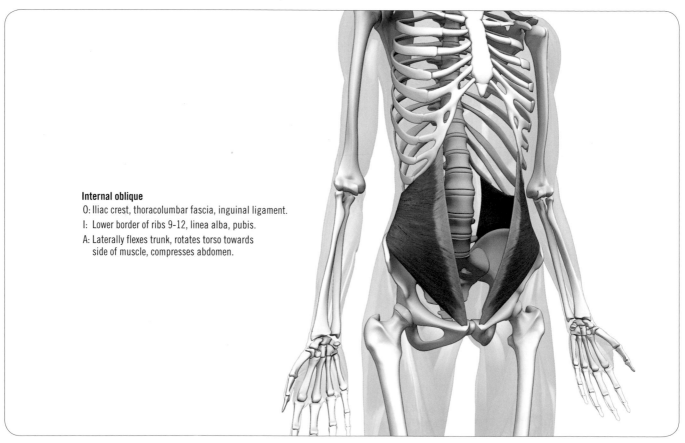

Internal oblique

O: Iliac crest, thoracolumbar fascia, inguinal ligament.

I: Lower border of ribs 9-12, linea alba, pubis.

A: Laterally flexes trunk, rotates torso towards side of muscle, compresses abdomen.

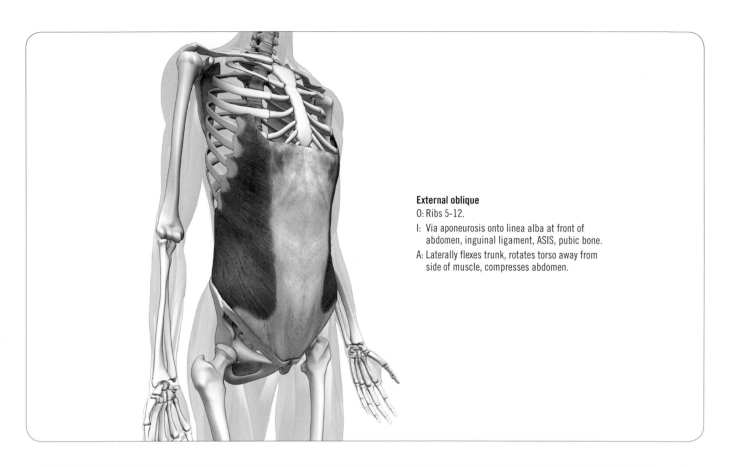

External oblique

O: Ribs 5-12.

I: Via aponeurosis onto linea alba at front of abdomen, inguinal ligament, ASIS, pubic bone.

A: Laterally flexes trunk, rotates torso away from side of muscle, compresses abdomen.

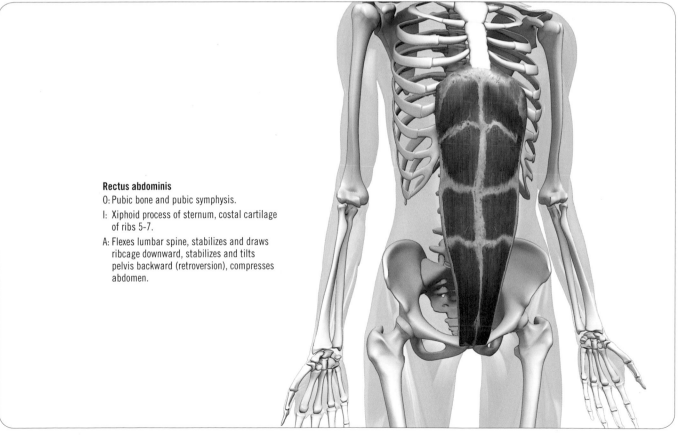

Rectus abdominis

O: Pubic bone and pubic symphysis.

I: Xiphoid process of sternum, costal cartilage of ribs 5-7.

A: Flexes lumbar spine, stabilizes and draws ribcage downward, stabilizes and tilts pelvis backward (retroversion), compresses abdomen.

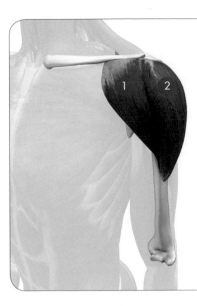

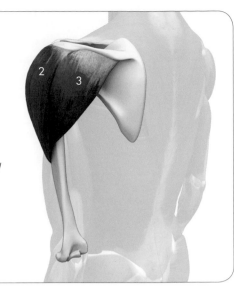

1 **Anterior deltoid**

O: Front and top of lateral third of clavicle.

I: Deltoid tuberosity on outer surface of humeral shaft.

A: Forward flexes and internally rotates humerus.

2 **Lateral deltoid**

O: Lateral border of acromion process of scapula.

I: Deltoid tuberosity on outer surface of humeral shaft.

A: Abducts humerus following initiation of movement by supraspinatus muscle of rotator cuff.

3 **Posterior deltoid**

O: Spine of scapula.

I: Deltoid tuberosity on outer surface of humeral shaft.

A: Extends and externally rotates humerus.

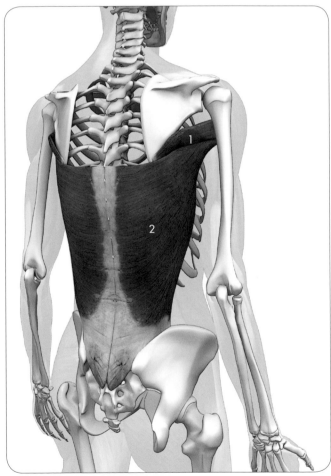

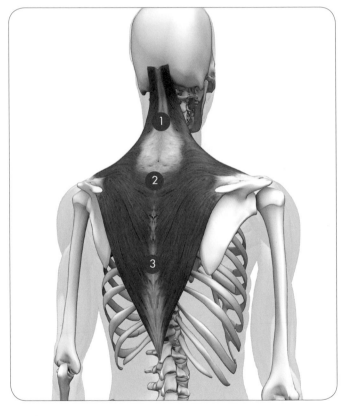

1 **Teres major**

O: Lower lateral border of scapula.

I: Bicipital groove of humerus.

A: Adducts and internally rotates humerus.

2 **Latissimus dorsi**

O: Thoracolumbar fascia, posterior portion of iliac crest, ribs 9-12, inferior border of scapula.

I: Bicipital groove of humerus.

A: Extends, adducts, and internally rotates humerus.

1 **Upper trapezius**

O: Occipital bone, ligamentum nuchae.

I: Upper border of spine of scapula.

A: Elevates (lifts) shoulder girdle, with lower trapezius rotates scapula to lift arm overhead.

2 **Middle trapezius**

O: Spinous processes of C7-T7.

I: Medial edge of acromion, posterior part of lateral third of clavicle.

A: Adducts (retracts) scapula.

3 **Lower trapezius**

O: Spinous processes of T8-12.

I: Medial edge of acromion, posterior part of lateral third of clavicle.

A: Depresses scapula, aids to hold body in arm balancing, with upper trapezius rotates scapula to lift arm overhead.

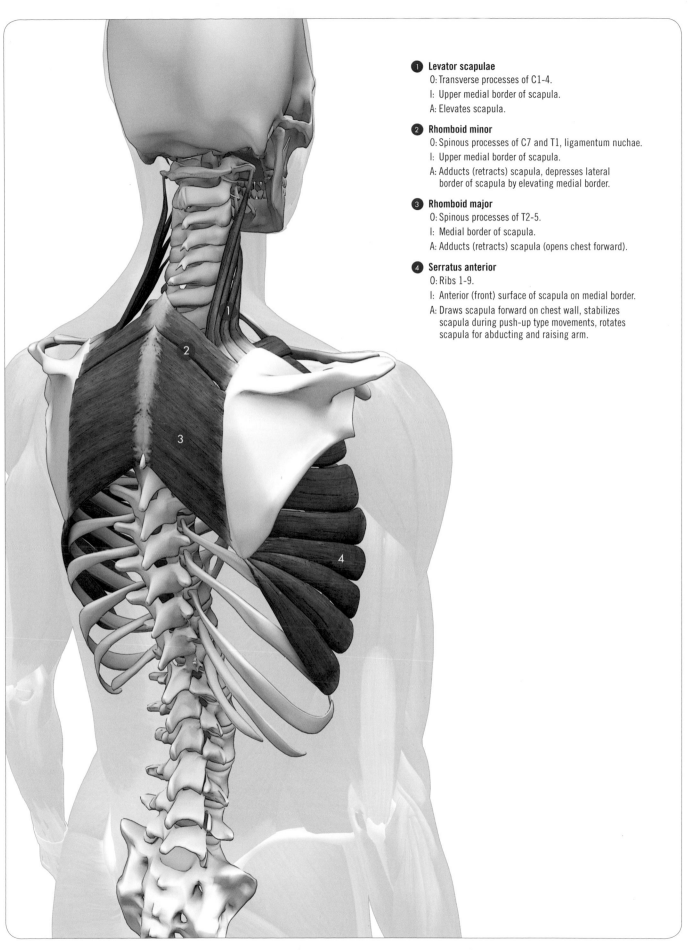

1 **Levator scapulae**

O: Transverse processes of C1-4.

I: Upper medial border of scapula.

A: Elevates scapula.

2 **Rhomboid minor**

O: Spinous processes of C7 and T1, ligamentum nuchae.

I: Upper medial border of scapula.

A: Adducts (retracts) scapula, depresses lateral border of scapula by elevating medial border.

3 **Rhomboid major**

O: Spinous processes of T2-5.

I: Medial border of scapula.

A: Adducts (retracts) scapula (opens chest forward).

4 **Serratus anterior**

O: Ribs 1-9.

I: Anterior (front) surface of scapula on medial border.

A: Draws scapula forward on chest wall, stabilizes scapula during push-up type movements, rotates scapula for abducting and raising arm.

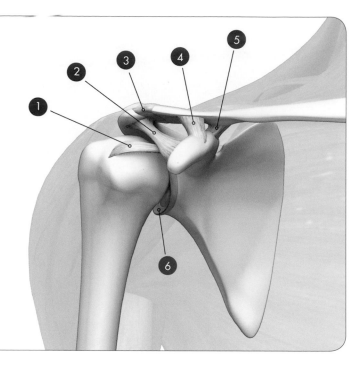

1. Coracohumeral ligament
2. Coracoacromial ligament
3. Acromioclavicular ligament
4. Trapezoid ligament
5. Conoid ligament
6. Glenoid labrum

1 Supraspinatus

O: Supraspinatus fossa of scapula.

I: Greater tuberosity of humerus.

A: Initiates abduction of humerus (raising arm to side), stabilizes head of humerus in socket of shoulder joint.

2 Subscapularis

O: Front surface of scapula in subscapular fossa.

I: Lesser tuberosity of humerus.

A: Internally rotates humerus, stabilizes head of humerus in socket of shoulder joint.

3 Teres minor

O: Upper part of lateral border of scapula.

I: Back and lower part of greater tuberosity of humerus.

A: Externally rotates humerus, stabilizes head of humerus in socket of shoulder joint.

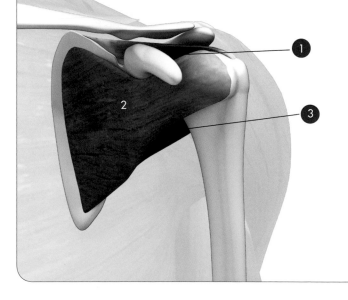

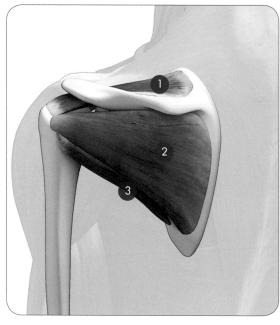

1 Supraspinatus

O: Supraspinatus fossa of scapula.

I: Greater tuberosity of humerus.

A: Initiates abduction of humerus (raising arm to side), stabilizes head of humerus in socket of shoulder joint.

2 Infraspinatus

O: Infraspinatus fossa of scapula.

I: Greater tuberosity of humerus.

A: Externally rotates shoulder.

3 Teres minor

O: Upper part of lateral border of scapula.

I: Back and lower part of greater tuberosity of humerus.

A: Externally rotates humerus, stabilizes head of humerus in socket of shoulder joint.

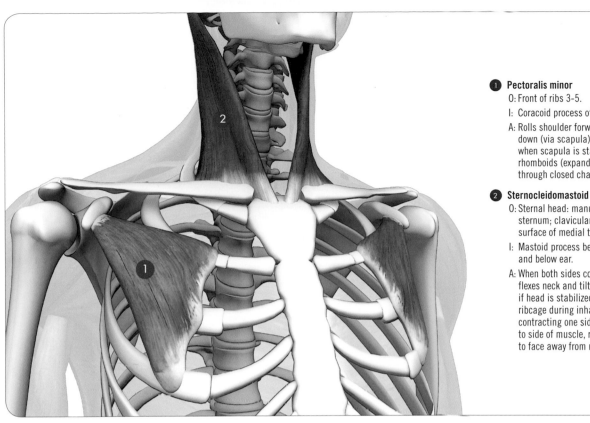

1 Pectoralis minor

O: Front of ribs 3-5.

I: Coracoid process of scapula.

A: Rolls shoulder forward and down (via scapula), lifts ribcage when scapula is stabilized by rhomboids (expands chest) through closed chain contraction.

2 Sternocleidomastoid

O: Sternal head: manubrium of sternum; clavicular head: upper surface of medial third of clavicle.

I: Mastoid process behind and below ear.

A: When both sides contract together flexes neck and tilts head forward; if head is stabilized, lifts upper ribcage during inhalation; contracting one side tilts head to side of muscle, rotates head to face away from muscle.

1 Pectoralis major

O: Sternocostal head: front of manubrium and body of sternum; clavicular head: medial half of clavicle.

I: Outer edge of bicipital groove on upper humerus.

A: Adducts and internally rotates humerus. Sternocostal head draws humerus down and across the body towards opposite hip. Clavicular head forward flexes and internally rotates the humerus, draws humerus across body towards opposite shoulder.

2 Coracobrachialis

O: Coracoid process of scapula.

I: Inner surface of humerus at mid-shaft.

A: Assists pectoralis in adduction of humerus and shoulder.

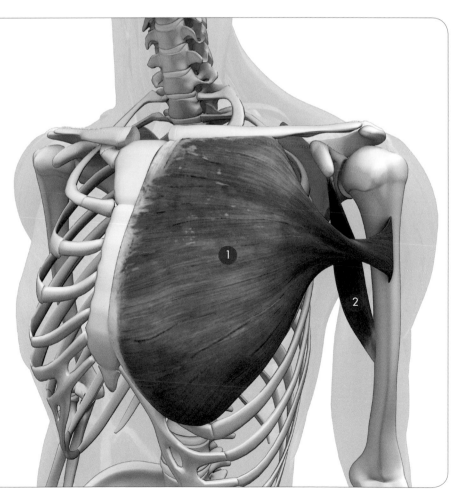

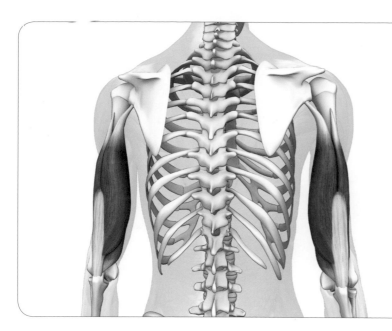

Triceps brachii

O: Long head from infraglenoid tubercle at bottom of shoulder socket; medial and lateral heads from posterior surface of humerus and intermuscular septum.

I: Olecranon process of ulna.

A: Extends elbow, long head moves arm back and adducts it.

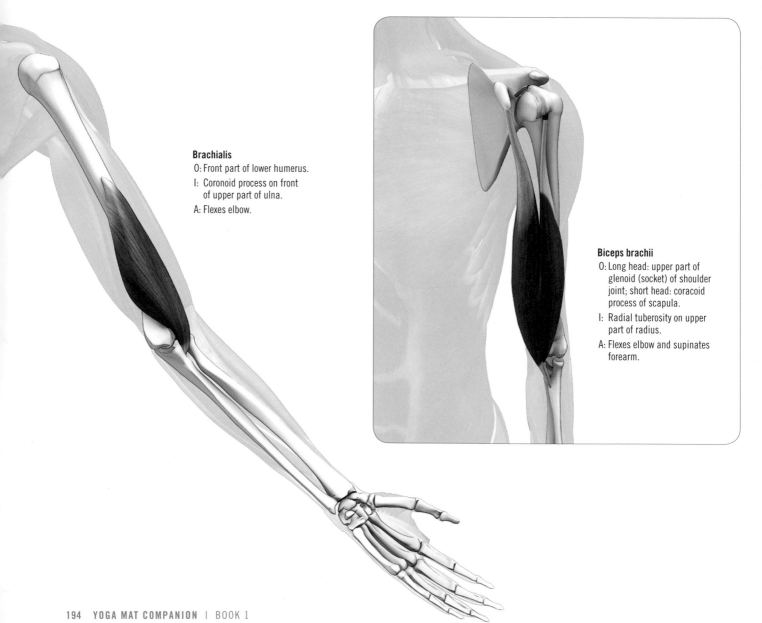

Brachialis

O: Front part of lower humerus.

I: Coronoid process on front of upper part of ulna.

A: Flexes elbow.

Biceps brachii

O: Long head: upper part of glenoid (socket) of shoulder joint; short head: coracoid process of scapula.

I: Radial tuberosity on upper part of radius.

A: Flexes elbow and supinates forearm.

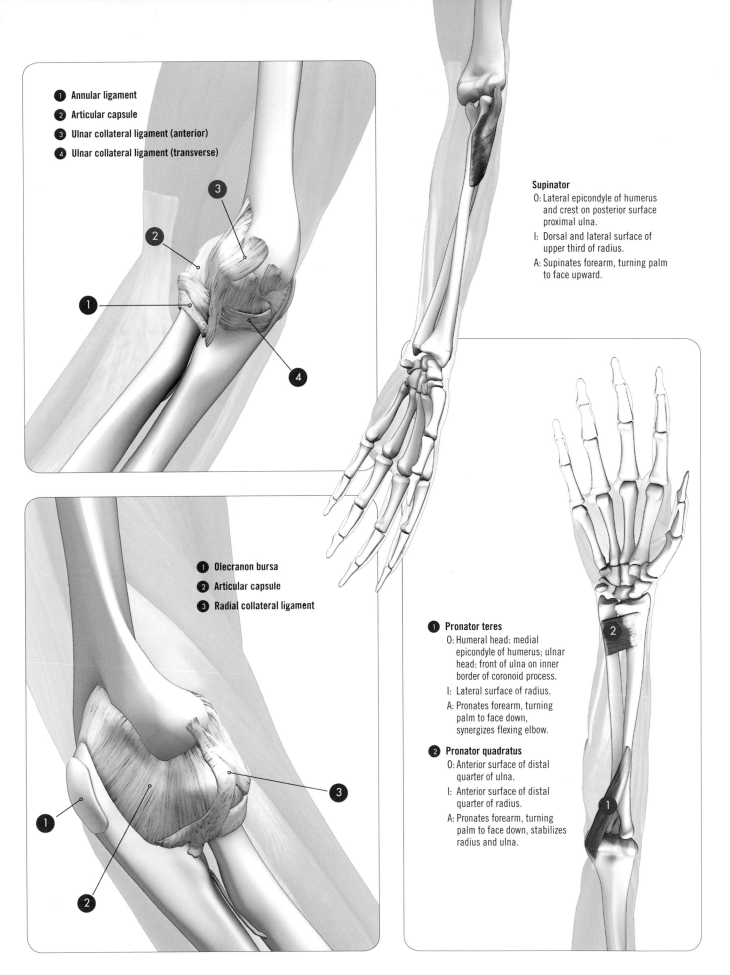

1 Annular ligament

2 Articular capsule

3 Ulnar collateral ligament (anterior)

4 Ulnar collateral ligament (transverse)

Supinator

O: Lateral epicondyle of humerus and crest on posterior surface proximal ulna.

I: Dorsal and lateral surface of upper third of radius.

A: Supinates forearm, turning palm to face upward.

1 Olecranon bursa

2 Articular capsule

3 Radial collateral ligament

1 Pronator teres

O: Humeral head: medial epicondyle of humerus; ulnar head: front of ulna on inner border of coronoid process.

I: Lateral surface of radius.

A: Pronates forearm, turning palm to face down, synergizes flexing elbow.

2 Pronator quadratus

O: Anterior surface of distal quarter of ulna.

I: Anterior surface of distal quarter of radius.

A: Pronates forearm, turning palm to face down, stabilizes radius and ulna.

1 **Flexor digitorum profundis**

O: Upper two thirds of anterior and medial surface of ulna and interosseous membrane (between radius and ulna).

I: Palmar (anterior) surface of distal phalanges of fingers.

A: Flexes distal phalanges, synergizes flexion of more proximal phalanges and wrist.

2 **Flexor pollicis longus**

O: Anterior surface of mid-shaft of radius, coronoid process of ulna, medial epicondyle.

I: Palmar (anterior) surface of distal phalanx of thumb.

A: Flexes thumb and synergizes flexion of wrist.

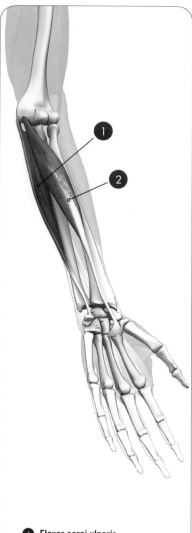

Flexor digitorum superficialis

O: Medial epicondyle, coronoid process of ulna, upper anterior border of radius.

I: Two slips of tendon insert onto either side of middle phalanges of four fingers.

A: Flexes middle phalanges of fingers, synergizes wrist flexion.

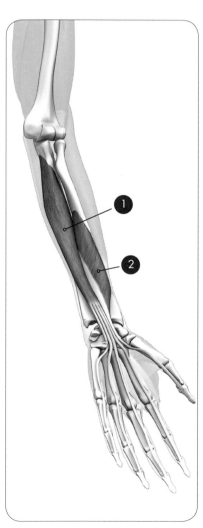

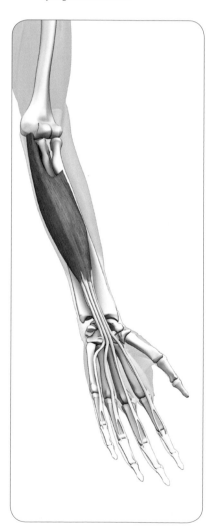

1 **Flexor carpi ulnaris**

O: Medial epicondyle of humerus, medial border and upper two thirds of ulna.

I: Pisiform bone of wrist, base of fifth metacarpal.

A: Flexes and adducts wrist, synergizes elbow flexion.

2 **Flexor carpi radialis**

O: Medial epicondyle of humerus.

I: Base of second metacarpal.

A: Flexes and abducts wrist, synergizes elbow flexion and pronation.

① Brachioradialis

O: Lateral supracondylar ridge of humerus.

I: Lower outside surface of radius, proximal to styloid process.

A: Flexes elbow.

② Extensor carpi radialis longus

O: Lateral supracondylar ridge of humerus.

I: Dorsal surface of base of second metacarpal.

A: Extends and abducts wrist.

③ Extensor carpi radialis brevis

O: Lateral epicondyle via common extensor tendon.

I: Dorsal surface of base of third metacarpal.

A: Extends and abducts wrist.

④ Extensor carpi ulnaris

O: Lateral epicondyle via common extensor tendon.

I: Base of fifth metacarpal.

A: Extends and adducts wrist.

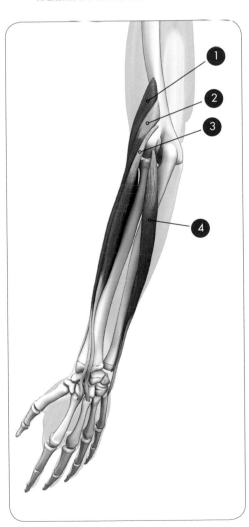

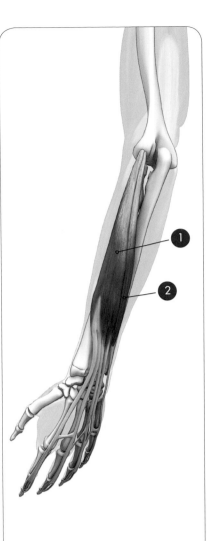

① Extensor digitorum

O: Lateral epicondyle via common extensor tendon.

I: Dorsal surfaces of phalanges of all four fingers.

A: Extends fingers, synergizes finger abduction away from midline.

② Extensor digiti minimi

O: Lateral epicondyle via common extensor tendon.

I: Combines with tendon of extensor digitorum to insert onto dorsum of little finger.

A: Extends little finger.

① Abductor pollicis longus

O: Posterior surface of ulna and radius covering middle third of bones, interosseous membrane.

I: Lateral surface of first metacarpal.

A: Extends and abducts thumb, synergist of forearm supination and wrist flexion.

② Extensor pollicis brevis

O: Posterior surface of distal radius, interosseous membrane.

I: Dorsal surface of base of proximal phalanx of thumb.

A: Extends thumb, synergizes wrist abduction.

③ Extensor pollicis longus

O: Posterior surface of middle third of ulna, interosseous membrane.

I: Dorsal surface at base of distal phalanx of thumb.

A: Extends thumb, synergizes wrist extension.

④ Extensor indicis

O: Posterior surface of distal ulna, interosseous membrane.

I: Dorsal aponeurosis of index finger, onto proximal phalanx.

A: Extends index finger.

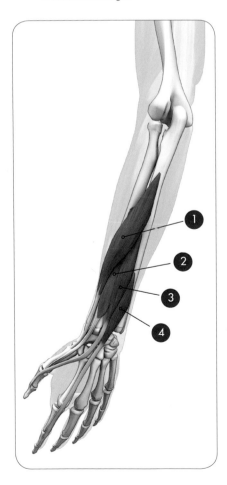

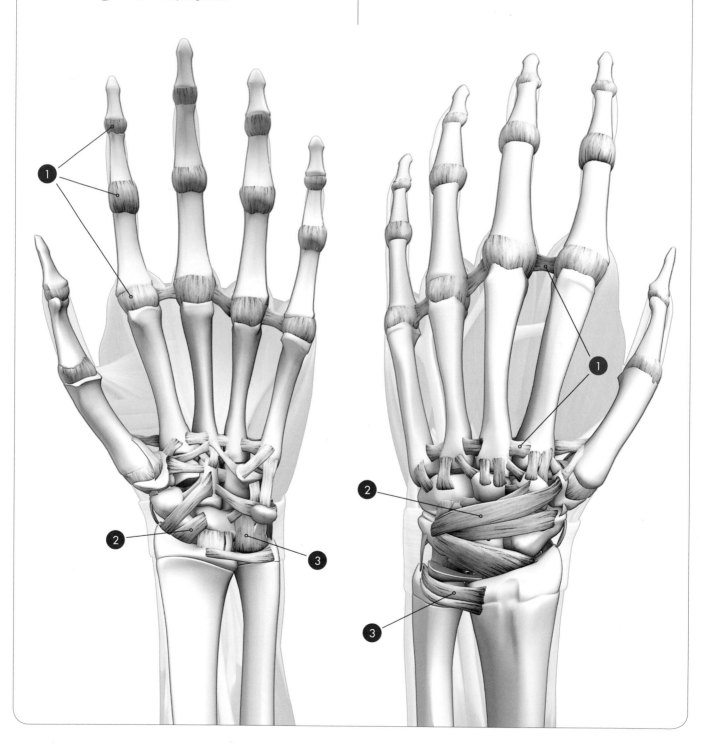

1 Metacarpophalangeal and interphalangeal joint capsules.

2 Palmar radiocarpal and intercarpal ligaments.

3 Palmar ulnocarpal ligament.

1 Transverse metacarpal ligaments.

2 Dorsal intercarpal ligaments.

3 Dorsal radioulnar ligament.

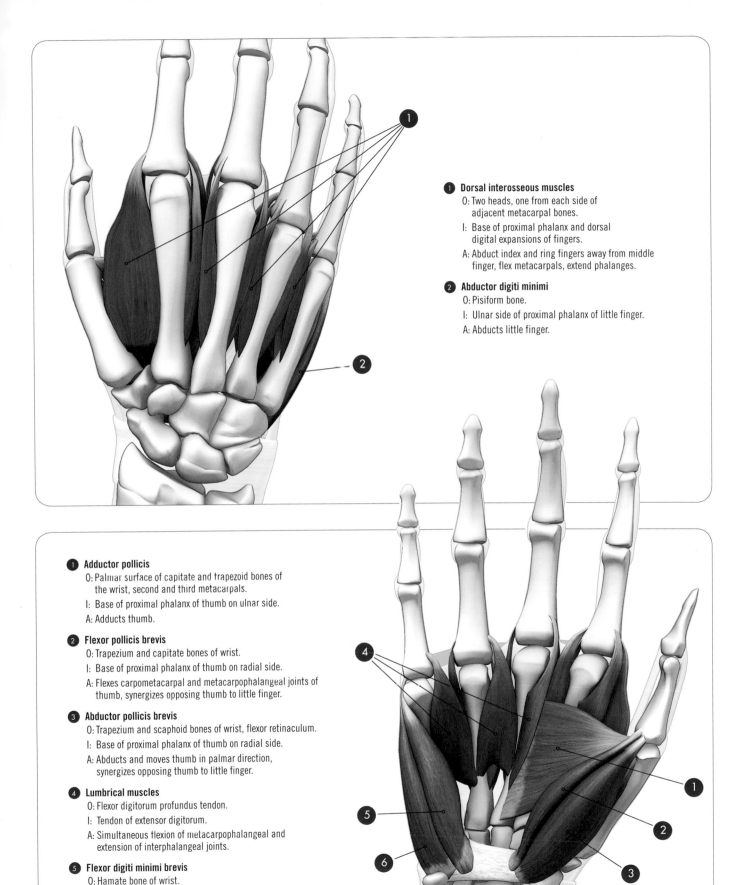

1 **Dorsal interosseous muscles**

O: Two heads, one from each side of adjacent metacarpal bones.

I: Base of proximal phalanx and dorsal digital expansions of fingers.

A: Abduct index and ring fingers away from middle finger, flex metacarpals, extend phalanges.

2 **Abductor digiti minimi**

O: Pisiform bone.

I: Ulnar side of proximal phalanx of little finger.

A: Abducts little finger.

1 **Adductor pollicis**

O: Palmar surface of capitate and trapezoid bones of the wrist, second and third metacarpals.

I: Base of proximal phalanx of thumb on ulnar side.

A: Adducts thumb.

2 **Flexor pollicis brevis**

O: Trapezium and capitate bones of wrist.

I: Base of proximal phalanx of thumb on radial side.

A: Flexes carpometacarpal and metacarpophalangeal joints of thumb, synergizes opposing thumb to little finger.

3 **Abductor pollicis brevis**

O: Trapezium and scaphoid bones of wrist, flexor retinaculum.

I: Base of proximal phalanx of thumb on radial side.

A: Abducts and moves thumb in palmar direction, synergizes opposing thumb to little finger.

4 **Lumbrical muscles**

O: Flexor digitorum profundus tendon.

I: Tendon of extensor digitorum.

A: Simultaneous flexion of metacarpophalangeal and extension of interphalangeal joints.

5 **Flexor digiti minimi brevis**

O: Hamate bone of wrist.

I: Base of proximal phalanx of little finger on ulnar side.

A: Flexes little finger.

6 **Abductor digiti minimi**

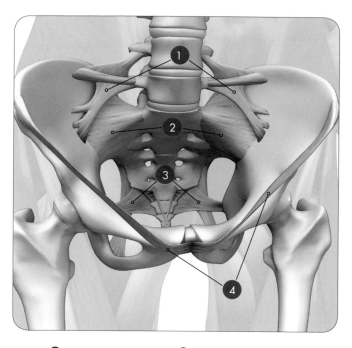

1 Iliolumbar ligament   3 Sacrospinous ligament

2 Sacroiliac ligament   4 Inguinal ligament

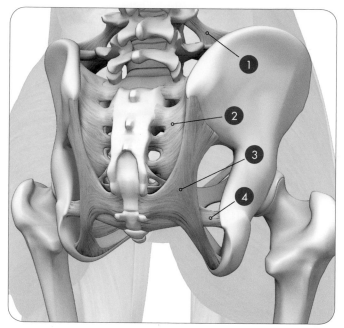

1 Iliolumbar ligament   3 Sacrotuberous ligament

2 Sacroiliac ligament   4 Sacrospinous ligament

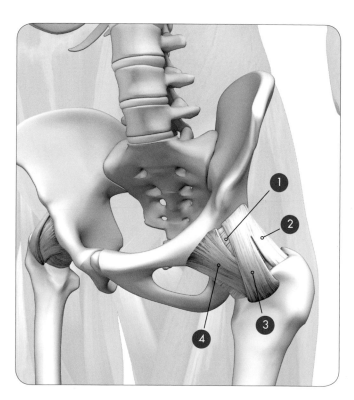

1 Zona orbicularis (hip capsule)   3 Anterior iliofemoral ligament

2 Lateral iliofemoral ligament   4 Pubofemoral ligament

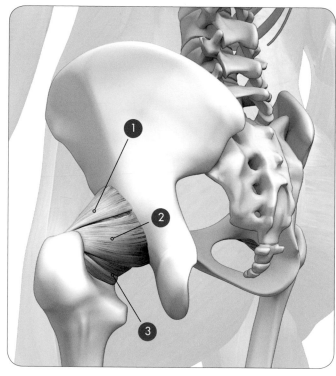

1 Lateral iliofemoral ligament   3 Zona orbicularis (hip capsule)

2 Ischiofemoral ligament

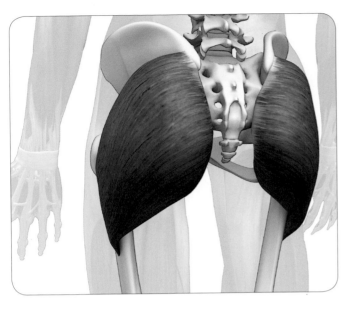

Gluteus maximus

O: Posterolateral surface of ilium and lateral surface of the sacrum.

I: Upper fibers onto iliotibial tract; lower fibers onto gluteal tuberosity.

A: Extends, externally rotates, and stabilizes hip.

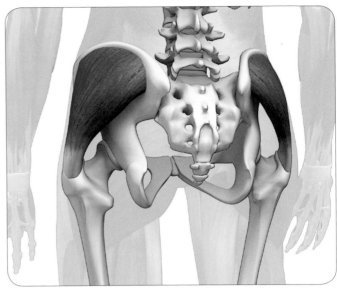

Gluteus medius

O: Outer surface of ilium.

I: Greater trochanter.

A: Abducts hip, anterior fibers internally rotate and flex hip, posterior fibers externally rotate and extend hip.

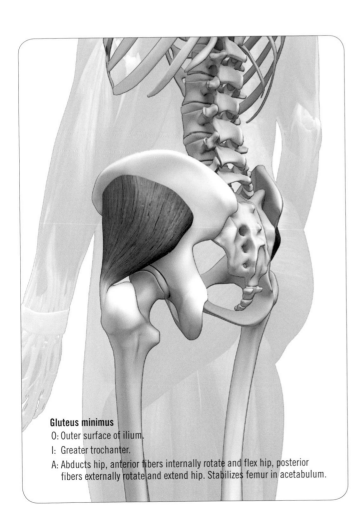

Gluteus minimus

O: Outer surface of ilium.

I: Greater trochanter.

A: Abducts hip, anterior fibers internally rotate and flex hip, posterior fibers externally rotate and extend hip. Stabilizes femur in acetabulum.

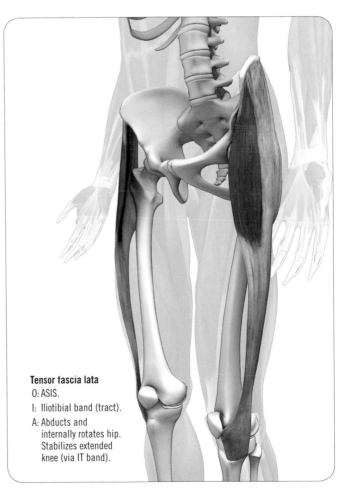

Tensor fascia lata

O: ASIS.

I: Iliotibial band (tract).

A: Abducts and internally rotates hip. Stabilizes extended knee (via IT band).

1 Piriformis

　　O: Posterior surface of sacrum.

　　I: Greater trochanter.

　　A: Externally rotates, abducts, extends, and stabilizes hip.

2 Superior gemellus

　　O: Ischial spine.

　　I: Greater trochanter.

　　A: Externally rotates and adducts hip.

3 Obturator internus

　　O: Obturator membrane and ischium.

　　I: Greater trochanter.

　　A: Externally rotates and adducts hip.

4 Inferior gemellus

　　O: Ischial tuberosity.

　　I: Greater trochanter.

　　A: Externally rotates and adducts hip.

5 Quadratus femoris

　　O: Ischial tuberosity.

　　I: Intertrochanteric crest.

　　A: Externally rotates and adducts hip.

6 Obturator externus

　　O: Obturator membrane and ischium.

　　I: Greater trochanter.

　　A: Externally rotates and adducts hip.

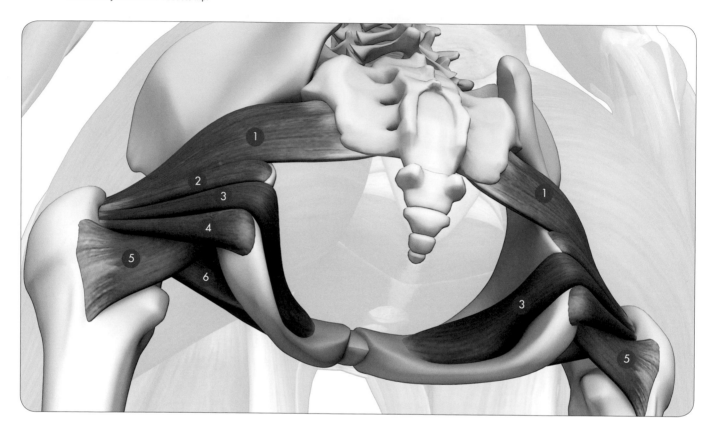

1 Psoas major

　　O: T12-L4 vertebral bodies and discs.

　　I: Lesser trochanter.

　　A: Flexes and externally rotates hip, stabilizes lumbar spine.

2 Iliacus

　　O: Inner surface of ilium.

　　I: Lesser trochanter.

　　A: Flexes and externally rotates hip, with psoas major tilts pelvis forward.

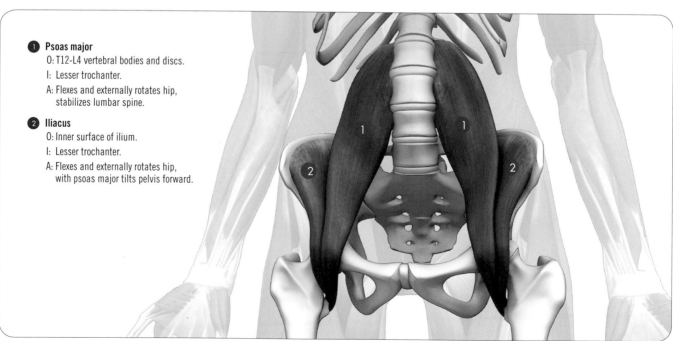

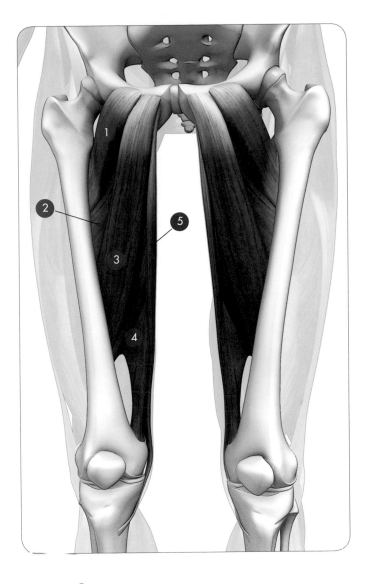

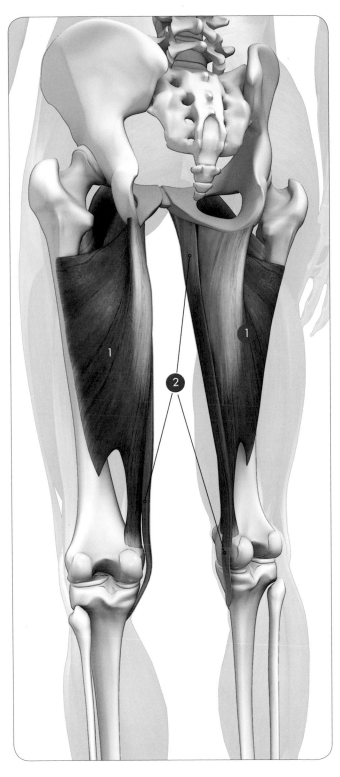

1 Pectineus
   O: Pubic bone.
   I: Linea aspera of femur.
   A: Adducts, externally rotates, and synergizes femur flexion.

2 Adductor brevis
   O: Pubic bone.
   I: Linea aspera of femur.
   A: Adducts and flexes femur, stabilizes pelvis.

3 Adductor longus
   O: Pubic bone.
   I: Linea aspera of femur.
   A: Adducts and flexes femur, stabilizes pelvis.

4 Adductor magnus
   O: Pubic bone and ischial tuberosity.
   I: Linea aspera and medial epicondyle of femur.
   A: Adducts, externally rotates, and extends femur.

5 Gracilis
   O: Pubic bone.
   I: Medial tibia.
   A: Adducts and flexes hip, flexes and internally rotates knee.

1 Adductor magnus

2 Gracilis

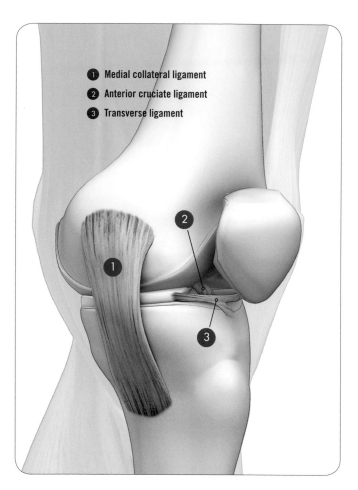

1 Medial collateral ligament
2 Anterior cruciate ligament
3 Transverse ligament

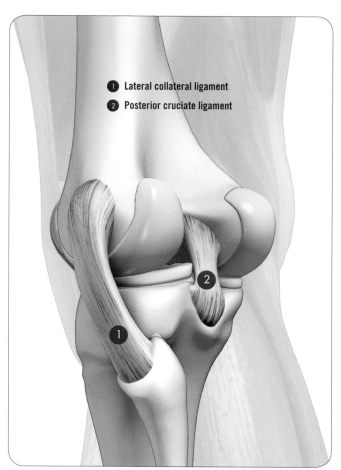

1 Lateral collateral ligament
2 Posterior cruciate ligament

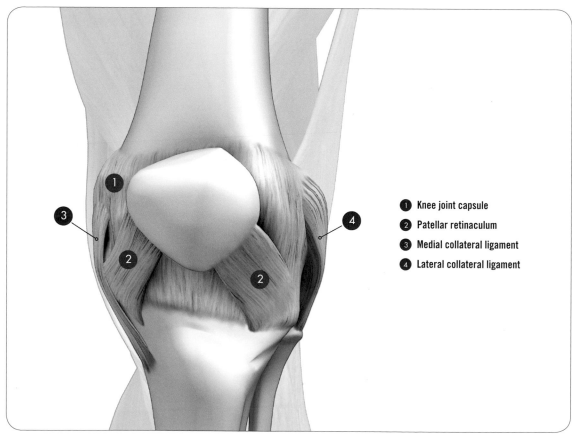

1 Knee joint capsule
2 Patellar retinaculum
3 Medial collateral ligament
4 Lateral collateral ligament

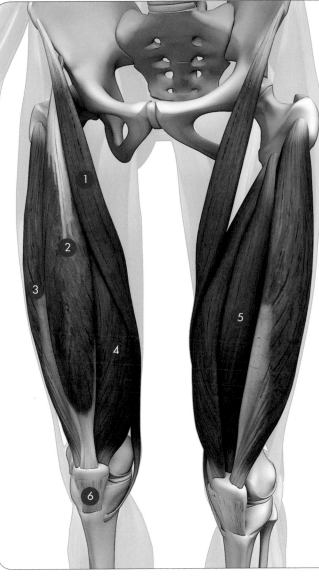

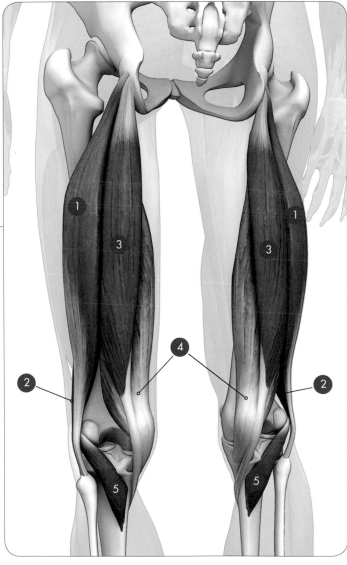

1. **Sartorius**
   O: ASIS.
   I: Pes anserinus of medial tibia.
   A: Flexes, abducts, and externally rotates hip; flexes and internally rotates knee.

2. **Rectus femoris**
   O: ASIS.
   I: Anterior tibia via patellar tendon.
   A: Flexes hip, tilts pelvis forward, extends knee.

3. **Vastus lateralis**
   O: Lateral femur.
   I: Anterior tibia via patellar tendon.
   A: Extends knee.

4. **Vastus medialis**
   O: Medial femur.
   I: Anterior tibia via patellar tendon.
   A: Extends knee.

5. **Vastus intermedius**
   O: Anterior femur.
   I: Anterior tibia via patellar tendon.
   A: Extends knee.

6. **Patellar tendon**

1. **Biceps femoris long head**
   O: Ischial tuberosity.
   I: Fibular head.
   A: Extends hip, flexes and externally rotates knee.

2. **Biceps femoris short head**
   O: Posterior surface of femur.
   I: Fibular head.
   A: Extends hip, flexes and externally rotates knee.

3. **Semitendinosus**
   O: Ischial tuberosity.
   I: Pes anserinus of medial tibia.
   A: Extends hip, flexes and internally rotates knee.

4. **Semimembranosus**
   O: Ischial tuberosity.
   I: Back of medial tibial condyle.
   A: Extends hip, flexes and internally rotates knee.

5. **Popliteus**
   O: Lateral femoral condyle.
   I: Posterior surface of tibia, below knee joint.
   A: Flexes and internally rotates knee.

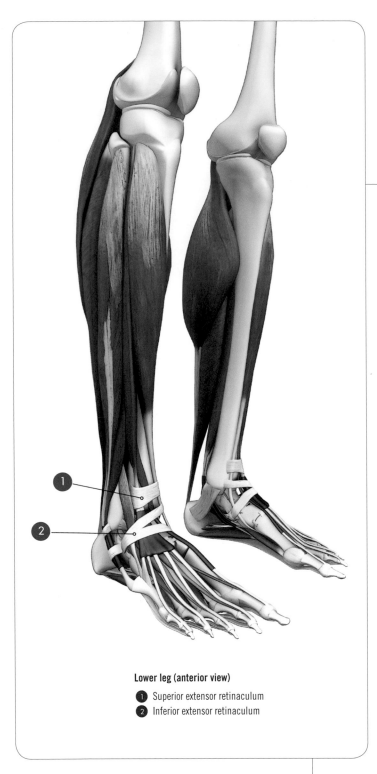

Lower leg (anterior view)

1. Superior extensor retinaculum
2. Inferior extensor retinaculum

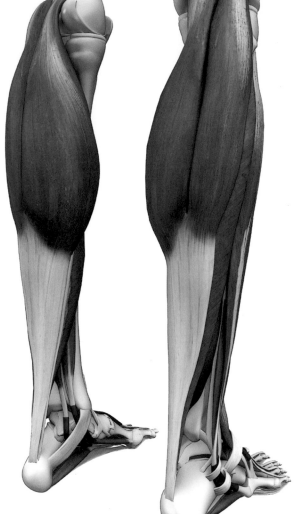

Lower leg (posterior view)

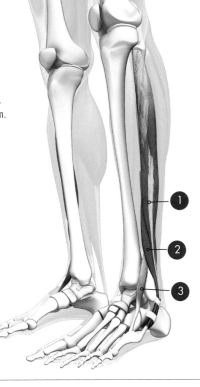

1 **Peroneus longus**

O: Head and proximal two thirds of lateral fibula.

I: Base of first metacarpal and medial cuneiform.

A: Plantar flexes ankle and everts subtalar joint, supports transverse arch of foot.

2 **Peroneus brevis**

O: Distal half of lateral surface of fibula, intermuscular membrane.

I: Base of fifth metatarsal.

A: Plantar flexes ankle and everts subtalar joint.

3 **Peroneus tertius**

O: Front of distal fibula.

I: Base of fifth metatarsal.

A: Dorsiflexes ankle and everts subtalar joint.

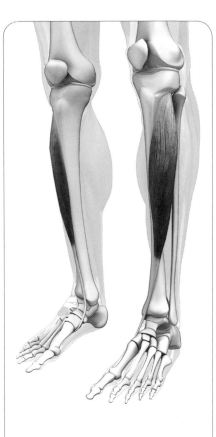

Tibialis anterior

O: Upper two thirds of anterior tibia and interosseous membrane.

I: Medial cuneiform, base of first metatarsal.

A: Dorsiflexes ankle, inverts subtalar joint.

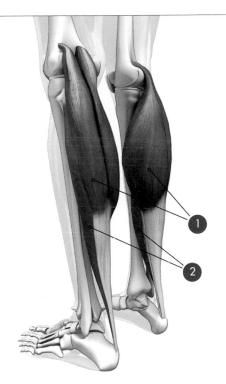

1 **Gastrocnemius**

O: Medial head from medial epicondyle of femur; lateral head from lateral epicondyle.

I: Calcaneous via Achilles tendon.

A: Plantar flexes and inverts ankle, flexes knee.

2 **Soleus**

O: Posterior surface of head and neck of fibula.

I: Calcaneous via Achilles tendon.

A: Plantar flexes ankle, inverts subtalar joint, and flexes knee.

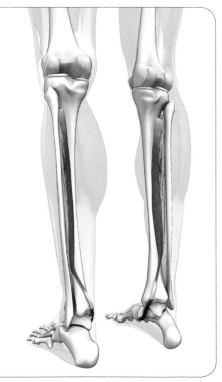

Tibialis posterior

O: Interosseous membrane between tibia and fibula.

I: Navicular, cuneiform bones, and second through fourth metatarsals.

A: Plantar flexes ankle, inverts subtalar joint, and supports longitudinal and transverse foot arches.

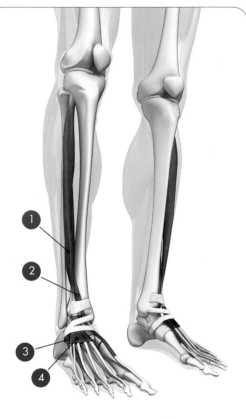

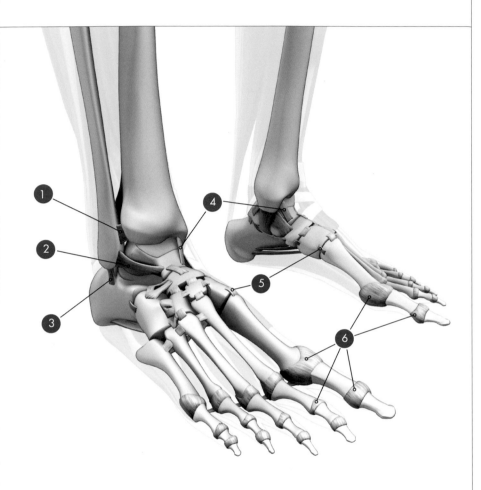

1. Anterior tibiofibular ligament
2. Anterior talofibular ligament
3. Calcaneofibular ligament
4. Anterior tibiotalar ligament
5. Dorsal metatarsal ligaments
6. Interphalangeal joint capsules

1. **Extensor digitorum longus**
   - O: Lateral tibial condyle, fibular head, interosseous membrane.
   - I: Dorsal aponeurosis and bases of the distal phalanges of second through fifth toes.
   - A: Dorsiflexes ankle, everts subtalar joint, and extends metatarsophalangeal and interphalangeal joints of toes.

2. **Extensor hallucis longus**
   - O: Medial surface of fibula, interosseous membrane.
   - I: Dorsal aponeurosis and base of distal phalanx of big toe.
   - A: Dorsiflexes ankle, everts subtalar joint, and extends big toe.

3. **Extensor digitorum brevis**
   - O: Dorsal surface of calcaneous.
   - I: Dorsal aponeurosis and bases of middle phalanges of second through fourth toes.
   - A: Extends metatarsophalangeal and proximal interphalangeal joints of second through fourth toes.

4. **Extensor tendons sheath**

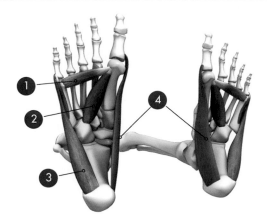

1 **Adductor hallucis (transverse head)**
   O: Metatarsophalangeal joints of third through fifth toes.
   I: Base of proximal phalanx of big toe via sesamoid.
   A: Adducts and flexes big toe, supports transverse foot arch.

2 **Adductor hallucis (oblique head)**
   O: Bases of second through fourth metatarsals,
      lateral cuneiform, and cuboid.
   I: Base of proximal phalanx of big toe via sesamoid.
   A: Adducts and flexes big toe, supports longitudinal foot arch.

3 **Abductor digiti minimi**
   O: Calcaneous, plantar aponeurosis.
   I: Base of proximal phalanx of little toe.
   A: Flexes metatarsophalangeal joint and abducts
      little toe, supports longitudinal foot arch.

4 **Abductor hallucis**
   O: Calcaneous, plantar aponeurosis.
   I: Base of proximal phalanx of big toe.
   A: Flexes and abducts big toe, supports longitudinal foot arch.

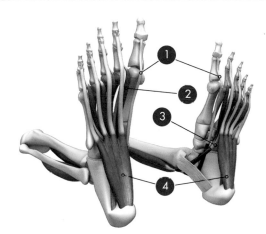

1 **Flexor hallucis longus**
   O: Posterior surface of fibula, interosseous membrane.
   I: Base of distal phalanx of big toe.
   A: Plantar flexes ankle, inverts subtalar joint, flexes
      big toe, supports longitudinal foot arch.

2 **Lumbrical muscles**
   O: Medial borders of flexor digitorum longus tendons.
   I: Dorsal aponeurosis of second through fifth toes.
   A: Flexes metatarsophalangeal and extends interphalangeal
      joints of second through fifth toes, adducts toe.

3 **Flexor digitorum longus**
   O: Posterior surface of tibia.
   I: Bases of distal phalanges of second through fifth toes.
   A: Plantar flexes ankle, inverts subtalar joint, plantar flexes toes.

4 **Flexor digitorum brevis**
   O: Calcaneous, plantar aponeurosis.
   I: Middle phalanges of second through fifth toes.
   A: Flexes toes, supports longitudinal foot arch.

1 Diaphragm

O: Lower margin of costal arch, posterior surface of xiphoid process of sternum, arcuate ligament of aorta, L1-3 vertebral bodies.

I: Central tendon.

A: Primary muscle of respiration, aids in compressing abdomen.

2 Intercostals

O: Internal intercostals from surface of upper margin of rib; external intercostals from lower margin of rib.

I: Internals insert on lower margin of next higher rib; externals insert on upper margin of next lower rib.

A: Internal intercostals lower ribs during exhalation; externals raise ribs during inhalation.

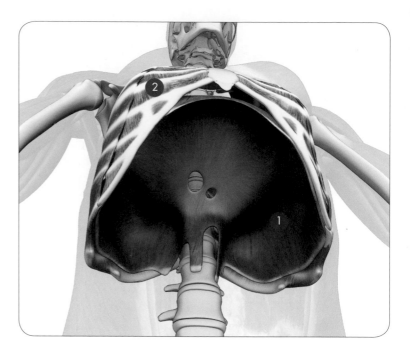

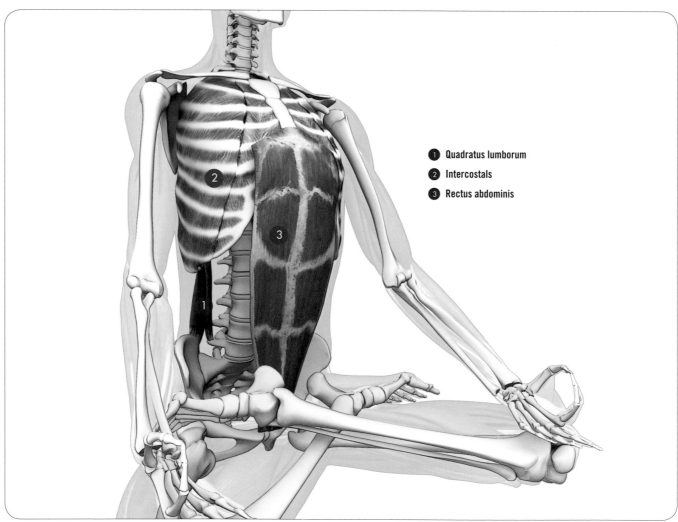

1 Quadratus lumborum

2 Intercostals

3 Rectus abdominis

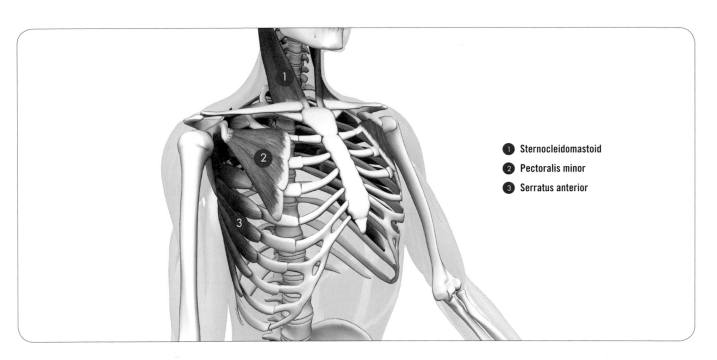

1. Sternocleidomastoid
2. Pectoralis minor
3. Serratus anterior

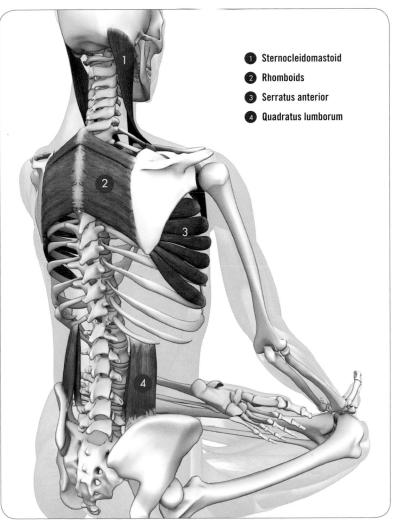

1. Sternocleidomastoid
2. Rhomboids
3. Serratus anterior
4. Quadratus lumborum

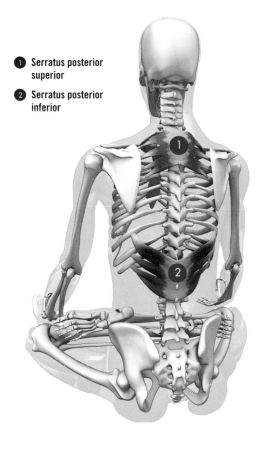

1. Serratus posterior superior
2. Serratus posterior inferior

INDEX OF MUSCLES AND LIGAMENTS

GLOSSARY OF TERMS

Abduction Moving away from the midline.

Accessory muscles of breathing Muscles that attach to the ribcage and thorax that can be used to augment the action of the diaphragm for inhalation and exhalation. These include the rhomboids, pectorals, quadratus lumborum, sternocleidomastoid, and intercostals (among others).

Active insufficiency A condition in which a muscle is shortened or lengthened to a point where it can no longer effectively move a joint. For example, in Kurmasana the hips are fully flexed and so the psoas muscle is shortened to a point where it cannot effectively flex the hips further. At such times, other parts of the body must be used for leverage, such as the arms under the knees.

Adduction Moving toward the midline.

Agonist The muscle that contracts to produce a certain action about a joint (sometimes referred to as the prime mover). For example, the brachialis contracts to flex the elbow joint.

Alveoli Sac-like spherical structures with thin membrane-like walls through which gas exchange occurs in the lungs.

Anatomy The study of the structure of living things. Musculoskeletal anatomy studies the bones, ligaments, muscles, and tendons.

Antagonist The muscle that opposes the action of the agonist muscle and produces the opposite action about a joint. For example, the hamstrings are the antagonists to the quadriceps for extending the knee.

Anteversion Tilting forward.

Aponeurosis A fibrous thickening of fascia that forms the attachment for muscles. For example, the abdominal muscles attach to the linea alba, an aponeurotic thickening at the front of the abdomen.

Appendicular skeleton Composed of the shoulder (pectoral girdle) and upper extremities and pelvis and lower extremities.

Asana Sanskrit term for body position in yoga (yogasana).

Autonomic nervous system Part of the nervous system that functions largely unconsciously to control breathing, heart rate, blood pressure, digestion, perspiration, and other functions. It is divided into the sympathetic (fight or flight) and parasympathetic (rest and digest) nervous systems.

Axial skeleton Composed of the skull, spine, and ribcage.

Bandha Sanskrit term referring to binding, locking, or stabilizing. Co-activating muscle groups can be used to form bandhas in yoga postures.

Biomechanics The application of mechanical physics to the body. For example, contracting the biceps flexes the elbow joint.

Carpals The bones of the wrist, including the scaphoid, lunate, triquetrum, hamate, capitate, trapezoid, and trapezium.

Center of gravity The center of an object's weight distribution and at which point an object is in balance.

Center of gravity projection An extension of the force of gravity downward and away from the body. For example, in Warrior III the center of gravity is projected out through the arms and the back leg, balancing the pose.

Chakra Wheel-like centers or concentrations of energy within the subtle body. They may correspond to collections of nerves such as the lumbosacral plexus (for the first and second chakras).

Closed chain contraction/movement The origin of the muscle moves and the insertion remains stationary. For example, the psoas contracts to flex the trunk in Trikonasana.

Co-contraction/co-activation Simultaneously contracting agonist and antagonist muscles to stabilize a joint. For example, co-activating the peroneus longus and brevis and the tibialis posterior muscles stabilizes the ankle joint.

Core muscles Composed of the transversus abdominis, internal and external obliques, rectus abdominis, erector spinae, psoas, gluteus maximus, and pelvic diaphragm.

Drishti Sanskrit term for focus of vision or gaze.

Eccentric contraction The muscle generates tension (contracts) while lengthening.

Erector spinae The group of three deep back muscles that run parallel to the spinal column, including the spinalis, longissimus, and iliocostalis muscles.

Eversion Rotating the sole of the foot (via the ankle) away from the midline of the body. This is associated with pronation (internal rotation) of the forefoot.

Extension Joint movement that increases space and distance between skeletal segments, bringing them farther apart.

Facilitated stretching A powerful method of stretching in which the muscle is first taken out to its full length and then contracted for several moments. This stimulates the Golgi tendon organ and produces the "relaxation response," causing the muscle to relax and lengthen. It is also known as PNF.

Fascia Connective tissue that surrounds, separates, and binds muscles to each other. This can also form an aponeurosis for muscle attachment.

Flexion Joint movement that decreases space between skeletal segments and draws them closer together.

Floating ribs Five pairs of ribs that articulate posteriorly with the vertebrae and attach to the costal cartilage anteriorly.

Forefoot The region of the foot distal to the midfoot. It is composed of the metatarsal and phalangeal bones (and their corresponding joints). Motion includes toe flexion and extension and deepening of the foot arches.

Glenohumeral joint Ball and socket synovial joint where the head (ball) of the humerus articulates with the glenoid fossa (socket) of the scapula.

Golgi tendon organ A sensory receptor located at the muscle-tendon junction that detects changes in tension. This information is conveyed to the central nervous system, which then signals the muscle to relax, providing "slack" in the muscle. This protects against the tendon being torn from the bone. The Golgi tendon organ is central to PNF or facilitated stretching.

Hindfoot Typically refers to the calcaneous and talus bones. The joint for the hindfoot is the subtalar joint, which is responsible for everting and inverting the foot. For example, the hindfoot is inverted in the back leg in Warrior I.

Iliotibial tract Fibrous fascial structure that runs on the outside of the thigh and blends into the lateral portion of the knee capsule. This forms the attachment for the tensor fascia lata and part of the gluteus maximus muscles.

Impingement Narrowing or encroachment of the space between two bones. It can cause inflammation and pain. For example, a nerve root can become impinged by a herniated intervertebral disc. You can also have impingement between the humeral head and the acromion, causing pain in the shoulder.

Insertion The distal site where a muscle attaches to a bone (via a tendon), usually farther from the midline of the body and more mobile than the muscle origin at its opposite end.

Inversion Rotating the sole of the foot towards the midline of the body (turning it inward). This is associated with supination (external rotation) of the forefoot.

Isometric contraction The muscle generates tension but does not shorten, and the bones do not move.

Isotonic contraction The muscle shortens while maintaining constant tension through a range of motion.

Kriya Sanskrit term for action or activity.

Leverage Creating a mechanical advantage based on the length of the lever. For example, placing the hand on the outside of the foot in Parivrtta Trikonasana uses the length of the arm for leverage to turn the body.

Line of action A line through which forces act or are directed within the body. For example, there is a line of action extending from the tips of the fingers to the heel in Utthita Parsvakonasana.

Metacarpals The intermediate region of the hand between the carpus (wrist) and the fingers, i.e., the five bones of the palms of the hands.

Midfoot The intermediate region of the foot between the hindfoot and forefoot. It is composed of the navicular, the cuboid, and three cuneiform bones. Motion includes contribution to supination and pronation of the forefoot.

Mudra Sanskrit term for seal; similar to a bandha. It is often performed with the hands by bringing the fingertips together in a specific way. Other mudras are created by combining bandhas throughout the body.

Muscle spindle A sensory receptor within the muscle belly that detects changes in length and tension in the muscle. This information is conveyed to the central nervous system which can then signal the muscle to contract to resist stretching. This reflex protects against tearing the muscle.

Open chain contraction/movement The insertion of the muscle moves and the origin remains stationary. For example, the deltoids contract to lift the arms in Warrior II.

Origin The proximal site where a muscle attaches to a bone (via a tendon), usually closer to the midline of the body and less mobile than the muscle insertion on the bone at its opposite end.

Parivrtta Revolving, twisted, or turning version of a pose. For example, Parivrtta Trikonasana is the revolving version of Trikonasana (Triangle Pose).

Pelvic girdle The ilium, ischium, pubic bones, and pubic symphysis.

Physiology The study of the functional processes of living things. Most physiological processes take place unconsciously but can be influenced by the conscious mind. Examples include breathing and facilitated stretching.

PNF Proprioceptive neuromuscular facilitation. Also known as *facilitated stretching*. (See facilitated stretching.)

Posterior kinetic chain Composed of a group of interconnecting ligaments, tendons, and muscles on the back of the body. Includes the hamstrings, gluteus maximus, erector spinae, trapezius, latissimus, and posterior deltoids.

Pranayama Yogic art of controlling the breath.

Prime mover The muscle that contracts to directly produce a desired movement. For example, the quadriceps contracts to extend the knee joint. The term is sometimes used interchangeably with 'agonist muscle.'

Radial deviation Tilting the hand toward the index-finger side or away from the midline of the body.

Reciprocal inhibition A phenomenon whereby the brain signals an agonist muscle to contract, and a simultaneous inhibitory signal is sent to the antagonist muscle, causing it to relax. This physiological process takes place unconsciously.

Retroversion Tilting backward.

Rotation Joint movement around a longitudinal axis. For example, we externally rotate the humerus bones (longitudinal axis) to turn the palms to face up in Savasana.

Scapulohumeral rhythm Simultaneous movements at the glenohumeral and scapulothoracic joints that function together to abduct and flex the shoulders. For example, scapulohumeral rhythm takes place when we raise the arms overhead in Urdhva Hastasana.

Shoulder girdle The clavicles and scapulae.

Synergist A muscle that assists and fine-tunes the action of the agonist or prime mover. It can be used to produce the same action, although generally not as efficiently. For example, the pectineus muscle synergizes the psoas in flexing the hip joint.

True ribs Seven pairs of ribs that articulate posteriorly with the vertebrae and anteriorly with the sternum.

Ulnar deviation Tilting the hand toward the little-finger side or midline of the body.

SANSKRIT PRONUNCIATION AND POSE INDEX

Sanskrit	Pronunciation	Pages
Adho Mukha Svanasana	[AH-doh MOO-kah shvah-NAHS-anna]	40
Ardha Uttanasana	[ARE-dah OOT-tan-AHS-ahna]	44, 50
Ardha Chandrasana	[ARE-dah chan-DRAHS-anna]	108, 114, 128
Ardha Matsyendrasana	[ARE-dah MOT-see-en-DRAHS-anna]	162
Baddha Konasana	[BAH-dah cone-NAHS-anna]	47, 72
Bakasana	[bahk-AHS-anna]	51
Bhujapidasana	[boo-jah-pi-dah-sana]	50
Chaturanga	[chaht-tour-ANG-ah]	36, 44, 46, 48, 50, 52
Dandasana	[don-DAHS-anna]	18, 42, 43, 46, 48, 52, 53
Dhanurasana	[don-your-AHS-anna]	49
Eka Pada Sarvangasana	[aa-KAH pah-DAH Sar-van-GAHS-anna]	53
Garudasana	[gah-rue-DAHS-anna]	160
Halasana	[hah-LAHS-anna]	52, 53
Janu Sirsasana	[JAH-new shear-SHAHS-anna]	47
Kurmasana	[koohr-MAH-sah-nah]	17–20, 47
Marichyasana III	[mar-ee-chee-AHS-anna]	49
Natarajasana	[not-ah-raj-AHS-anna]	21
Parivrtta Ardha Chandrasana	[par-ee-vrt-tah are-dah chan-DRAHS-anna]	146, 174
Parivrtta Parsvakonasana	[par-ee-vrt-tah parsh-vah-cone-AHS-anna]	15, 45, 140, 146
Parivrtta Trikonasana	[par-ee-vrit-tah trik-cone-AHS-anna]	17, 45, 114, 134, 146, 148
Parsva Bakasana	[PARSH-vah bahk-AHS-anna]	51
Parsva Halasana	[PARSH-vah hah-LAHS-anna]	53
Parsvottanasana	[pars-VOH-tahn-AS-ahna]	9, 45, 114, 120
Paschimottanasana	[POSH-ee-moh-tan-AHS-anna]	46, 47, 66
Pincha Mayurasana	[pin-cha my-your-AHS-anna]	51
Prasarita Padottanasana	[pra-sa-REE-tah pah-doh-tahn-AHS-anna]	17, 19, 45, 154, 160
Purvottanasana	[purvo-tan AHS-Ahna]	49

Sarvangasana	[sar-van-GAHS-anna]	52
Savasana	[shah-VAHS-anna]	4, 50, 52, 53, 169
Setu Bandha	[SET-too BAHN-dah]	48, **168**, 169
Sirsasana	[shir-SHAHS-anna]	51
Surya Namaskar	[sur-YAH-nah mass-KAR]	44, 46
Tadasana	[tah-DAS-anna]	32, 42, 44, 46, 50, **56**, 71, 87, 116, 127
Triang Mukhaikapada Paschimottanasana	[tree-AWN-guh moo-KA-eh-ka-paw-duh POSH-ee -moh tun AWS ah-nah]	47
Upavistha Konasana	[oo-pah-VEESH-tah cone-AHS-anna]	47
Urdhva Dhanurasana	[OORD-vah don-your-AHS-anna]	48, 49
Urdhva Hastasana	[oord-vah hahs-TAHS-anna]	44, 50, 56
Urdhva Mukha Svanasana	[OORD-vah MOO-kah shvon-AHS-anna]	**38**
Utkatasana	[OOT-kah-TAHS-anna]	9, **82**
Uttanasana	[OOT-tan-AHS-ahna]	7, 34, 36, 44, 45, 50, **64**
Utthita Hasta Padangusthasana	[oo-TEE-tah - ha-sta-pah-don-GOO-stah-sa-na]	**76**
Utthita Parsvakonasana	[oo-TEE-tah parsh-vah-cone-AHS-anna]	7, 8, 45, **102**, 108, 174, 185
Utthita Trikonasana	[oo-TEE-tah trik-cone-AHS-anna]	6, **88**
Viparita Karani	[vip-par-ee-tah car-AHN-ee]	**169**
Virabhadrasana I	[veer-ah-bah-DRAHS-anna]	8, **120**
Virabhadrasana II	[veer-ah-bah-DRAHS-anna]	**94**, 103, 108, 120
Virabhadrasana III	[veer-ah-bah-DRAHS-anna]	94, **128**
Vrksasana	[vrik-SHAHS-anna]	**70**, 84

Other Sanskrit Terms	**Pronunciation**	**Pages**
Asana	[AHS-anna]	214
Ashtanga	[UHSSH-TAWN-gah]	52
Bandha	[bahn-dah]	214
Chakra	[CHUHK-ruh]	1, 48, 50, 52, 112, 128
Drishti	[dr-ISH-tee]	4
Hatha	[huh-tuh]	1, 4
Jalandhara Bandha	[jah-lahn-DHA-rah bahn-dah]	53
Kriya	[kr-EE-yah]	17
Mudra	[MOO-drah]	216
Mula Bandha	[moo-lah bahn-dah]	9, 87
Namasté	[nah-moss-te (*te* rhymes with *day*)]	114, 116, 119
Pranayama	[PRAH-nah-yama]	31
Udyana Bandha	[oo-dee-YAH-nah BAHN-dah]	——
Ujjayi	[oo-jy (*jy* rhymes with *pie*)-ee]	27, 30, 103
Vinyasa	[vin-YAH-sah]	27
Yoga	[YO-gah]	——

ENGLISH POSE INDEX

CONTRIBUTORS

CHRIS MACIVOR—a self-taught computer expert and digital artist—is the Technical Director for Bandha Yoga and Illustrator of the bestselling series, *The Key Muscles of Yoga* and *The Key Poses of Yoga*. He is a graduate of Etobicoke School of the Arts, Sheridan College, and Seneca College. With a background in dance and traditional art, as well as computer graphics and animation, Chris considers himself to be equally artistic and technical in nature. Working with Dr. Long on the Scientific Keys book series, he has digitally reproduced the biomechanical perfection of the human body. With a keen eye for subtle lighting and a passion for excellence in his art, Chris successfully brings his imagery to life.

KURT LONG, BFA, is an award-winning fine artist and anatomical illustrator who contributed the front and back cover illustrations. He is a graduate of the University of Pennsylvania and has studied at the Pennsylvania Academy of Fine Arts and the Art Students League of New York. Kurt resides in Philadelphia with his wife and two sons. For information on commissions and to see more of his work, go to www.KurtLong.net.

STEWART THOMAS contributed the Sanskrit calligraphy and the special hand-painted border for the Bandha Yoga Codex. He is an award-winning artist, calligrapher, printmaker and designer. A graduate of Haverford College and the University of the Arts in Philadelphia, he serves as Creative Director of Florida's Eden, a regional alliance working for a sustainable future for North Florida, and produces art at his own Palmstone Studio (www.palmstone.com).

ERYN KIRKWOOD, MA, RYT 200, graduated from Carleton University with a Master's Degree in English Literature. She left a corporate career as Managing Editor at the Canadian Medical Association to dedicate her life to the study, practice, and teaching of yoga. Eryn is the Chief Editor at Bandha Yoga and maintains an award-winning Blog. She offers alignment-focused yoga classes in Ottawa, Canada, and can be reached at www.BarrhavenYoga.com.

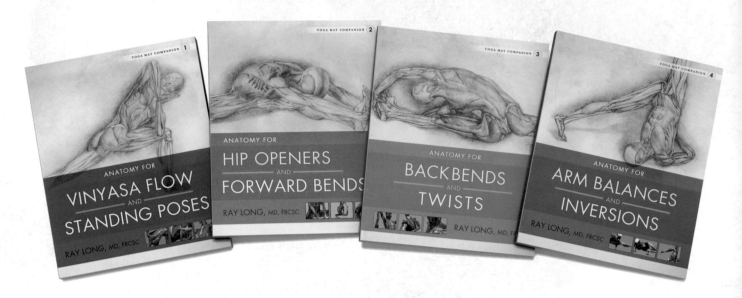

ALSO FROM BANDHA YOGA

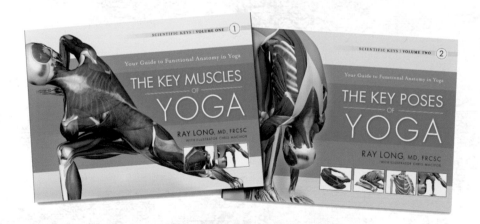

www.BandhaYoga.com